HERBAL TINCTURES FOR SPECIFIC AILMENTS

A HOLISTIC RECIPE BOOK

BY: TANYA SMITH

WELCOME TO "HERBAL TINCTURES FOR SPECIFIC AILMENTS: A HOLISTIC RECIPE BOOK"! THIS GUIDE WILL INTRODUCE YOU TO THE WONDERFUL WORLD OF HERBAL TINCTURES AND HOW TO CREATE TARGETED REMEDIES FOR VARIOUS AILMENTS AND SPECIFIC BODY SECTIONS. EXPLORE THE HEALING POTENTIAL OF NATURE AS WE DELVE INTO THE RECIPES THAT HARNESS THE POWER OF HERBS TO SUPPORT YOUR OVERALL WELL-BEING.

TABLE OF CONTENTS

CHAPTER 1: <u>UNDERSTANDING HERBAL TINCTURES</u>

CHAPTER 2: <u>HERBAL TINCTURES FOR AILMENTS</u>

CHAPTER 3: HERBAL TINCTURES FOR SPECIFIC BODY SECTIONS

- HEAD AND SINUSES

- THROAT AND RESPIRATORY SYSTEM

- HEART AND CIRCULATORY SYSTEM

- DIGESTIVE SYSTEM

- MUSCLES AND JOINTS

- SKIN AND HAIR

CHAPTER 4: RECIPES FOR SPECIFIC AILMENTS AND BODY SECTIONS

4.1 IMMUNE SYSTEM SUPPORT

- ELDERBERRY ELIXIR FOR COLD AND FLU

- ECHINACEA AND GOLDENSEAL BLEND FOR IMMUNE BOOST

4.2 DIGESTIVE HEALTH

- PEPPERMINT AND GINGER DIGESTIVE TONIC

- DANDELION AND BURDOCK BITTERS FOR DIGESTIVE SUPPORT

4.3 RESPIRATORY HEALTH

- MULLEIN AND MARSHMALLOW ROOT SYRUP FOR COUGH RELIEF

- THYME & EUCALYPTUS RESPIRATORY TONIC

4.4 SLEEP AND RELAXATION

- LAVENDER AND CHAMOMILE SLEEP AID

- VALERIAN AND PASSIONFLOWER CALMING ELIXIR

4.5 ENERGY AND VITALITY

- GINSENG AND MACA ENERGIZING TINCTURE

- NETTLE AND ASHWAGANDHA REVITALIZING BLEND

4.6 STRESS AND ANXIETY RELIEF

- LEMON BALM AND SKULLCAP STRESS-RELIEVING ELIXIR

- HOLY BASIL AND ASHWAGANDHA ADAPTOGEN TINCTURE

CONCLUSION: EMBRACING HOLISTIC WELLNESS WITH HERBAL TINCTURES

- BRINGING HOLISTIC WELLNESS INTO YOUR DAILY ROUTINE

- TIPS FOR SOURCING HIGH-QUALITY HERBS

- INCORPORATING HERBAL TINCTURES INTO A HEALTHIER LIFESTYLE

BY EXPLORING THIS RECIPE BOOK AND CRAFTING YOUR OWN HERBAL TINCTURES, YOU'LL BE ON YOUR WAY TO ENHANCING YOUR WELL-BEING NATURALLY BY HARNESSING THE POWER OF HERBS. REMEMBER TO CONSULT WITH A HEALTHCARE PROFESSIONAL BEFORE INCORPORATING HERBAL REMEDIES INTO YOUR ROUTINE, PARTICULARLY IF YOU HAVE ANY PRE-EXISTING MEDICAL CONDITIONS OR ARE TAKING MEDICATIONS.

GET READY TO EMBARK ON AN EMPOWERING JOURNEY TO HOLISTIC WELLNESS USING THE POTENT HEALING CAPACITY OF HERBAL TINCTURES!

CHAPTER 1

HERBAL TINCTURES ARE CONCENTRATED LIQUID EXTRACTS MADE FROM HERBS. THEY ARE CREATED BY SOAKING HERBS IN ALCOHOL OR A MIXTURE OF ALCOHOL AND WATER, ALLOWING THE ACTIVE COMPOUNDS TO BE EXTRACTED INTO THE LIQUID. THE ALCOHOL ACTS AS A SOLVENT, DRAWING OUT THE MEDICINAL PROPERTIES OF THE HERBS. TINCTURES ARE KNOWN FOR THEIR HIGH POTENCY AND ABILITY TO PRESERVE THE THERAPEUTIC PROPERTIES OF HERBS FOR AN EXTENDED PERIOD. THEY ARE COMMONLY USED IN HOLISTIC AND TRADITIONAL MEDICINE PRACTICES FOR THEIR HEALTH BENEFITS.

THERE ARE SEVERAL BENEFITS ASSOCIATED WITH USING HERBAL TINCTURES:

1. **HIGH POTENCY**: TINCTURES ARE HIGHLY CONCENTRATED EXTRACTS, MAKING THEM MORE POTENT THAN OTHER HERBAL PREPARATIONS SUCH AS TEAS OR CAPSULES. THIS ALLOWS FOR A MORE POTENT AND QUICKER ABSORPTION OF THE MEDICINAL COMPOUNDS.

2. **LONG SHELF LIFE**: TINCTURES TYPICALLY HAVE A LONG SHELF LIFE, OFTEN MAINTAINED FOR SEVERAL YEARS. THE ALCOHOL USED IN THE EXTRACTION PROCESS ACTS AS A PRESERVATIVE, HELPING TO PREVENT THE GROWTH OF BACTERIA OR FUNGI.

3. **<u>QUICK ABSORPTION</u>**: TINCTURES ARE TAKEN ORALLY, ALLOWING FOR RAPID ABSORPTION INTO THE BLOODSTREAM THROUGH THE MUCOUS MEMBRANES IN THE MOUTH. THIS QUICK ABSORPTION CAN LEAD TO FASTER AND MORE NOTICEABLE EFFECTS.

4. **<u>CUSTOMIZABLE DOSING</u>**: THE LIQUID FORM OF TINCTURES ALLOWS FOR EASY AND CUSTOMIZABLE DOSING. IT IS SIMPLE TO ADJUST THE DOSE BASED ON INDIVIDUAL NEEDS OR THE RECOMMENDED DOSAGE PROVIDED BY A HEALTHCARE PROFESSIONAL.

5. **<u>VERSATILITY</u>**: TINCTURES CAN BE MADE FROM A WIDE VARIETY OF HERBS, PROVIDING ACCESS TO A WIDE RANGE OF MEDICINAL PROPERTIES. THIS ALLOWS INDIVIDUALS TO TARGET SPECIFIC HEALTH CONCERNS OR COMBINE MULTIPLE HERBS FOR A SYNERGISTIC EFFECT.

6. **<u>CONVENIENCE</u>**: TINCTURES ARE EASY TO CARRY AND USE ON-THE-GO. THEY CAN BE CONVENIENTLY STORED IN SMALL DROPPER BOTTLES AND TAKEN ORALLY WHENEVER NEEDED.

7. **<u>ENHANCED EXTRACTION</u>**: ALCOHOL-BASED TINCTURES ARE PARTICULARLY EFFECTIVE AT EXTRACTING BOTH WATER-SOLUBLE AND ALCOHOL-SOLUBLE COMPOUNDS FROM HERBS, ENSURING THAT A BROADER RANGE OF ACTIVE CONSTITUENTS IS CAPTURED IN THE FINAL PRODUCT.

IT IS IMPORTANT TO NOTE THAT WHILE HERBAL TINCTURES CAN OFFER POTENTIAL HEALTH BENEFITS, IT IS ADVISABLE TO CONSULT WITH A HEALTHCARE PROFESSIONAL OR A QUALIFIED HERBALIST BEFORE STARTING ANY HERBAL REGIMEN.

PREPARING HERBAL TINCTURES AT HOME REQUIRES A FEW BASIC STEPS. HERE'S A GENERAL GUIDE TO GET YOU STARTED:

1. **<u>CHOOSE YOUR HERBS</u>**: SELECT THE HERBS YOU WANT TO USE BASED ON THEIR MEDICINAL PROPERTIES AND YOUR SPECIFIC NEEDS. IT'S IMPORTANT TO USE HIGH-QUALITY, ORGANIC HERBS FOR BEST RESULTS.

2. **<u>GATHER SUPPLIES</u>**: YOU'LL NEED THE FOLLOWING ITEMS:

- DRIED HERBS

- ALCOHOL (SUCH AS VODKA, BRANDY, OR RUM) WITH AT LEAST 40% ALCOHOL CONTENT

- GLASS JAR WITH A TIGHT-FITTING LID

- CHEESECLOTH OR FINE MESH STRAINER

- AMBER GLASS BOTTLES WITH DROPPER CAPS FOR STORAGE

3. **<u>PREPARE THE HERBS</u>**: IF NEEDED, CHOP OR GRIND THE DRIED HERBS INTO SMALLER PIECES TO INCREASE THE SURFACE AREA FOR EXTRACTION. THIS STEP IS OPTIONAL BUT CAN HELP IMPROVE THE EXTRACTION PROCESS.

4. **<u>COMBINE HERBS AND ALCOHOL</u>:** PLACE THE HERBS IN THE GLASS JAR, FILLING IT ABOUT ONE-THIRD TO HALFWAY. POUR ENOUGH ALCOHOL OVER THE HERBS TO COMPLETELY COVER THEM. ENSURE THAT THE HERB-TO-ALCOHOL RATIO IS APPROPRIATE, AS SOME HERBS MAY REQUIRE A HIGHER ALCOHOL CONCENTRATION FOR EFFECTIVE EXTRACTION.

5. **<u>SEAL AND SHAKE</u>:** CLOSE THE JAR TIGHTLY AND GIVE IT A GOOD SHAKE TO EVENLY MIX THE HERBS AND ALCOHOL. MAKE SURE THE HERBS ARE COMPLETELY SUBMERGED IN THE LIQUID.

6. **<u>MACERATE</u>**: PLACE THE SEALED JAR IN A COOL, DARK PLACE, LIKE A CUPBOARD OR PANTRY. LEAVE IT THERE FOR AT LEAST 4 TO 6 WEEKS FOR MACERATION. DURING THIS TIME, SHAKE THE JAR OCCASIONALLY TO PROMOTE EXTRACTION.

7. **<u>STRAIN THE TINCTURE</u>**: AFTER THE MACERATION PERIOD, STRAIN THE LIQUID USING A CHEESECLOTH OR FINE MESH STRAINER. SQUEEZE OUT AS MUCH LIQUID AS POSSIBLE FROM THE HERBS. YOU CAN REPEAT THIS PROCESS FOR A CLEANER AND MORE REFINED TINCTURE.

8. **<u>STORE AND LABEL</u>**: TRANSFER THE STRAINED TINCTURE INTO AMBER GLASS BOTTLES WITH DROPPER CAPS FOR STORAGE. LABEL EACH BOTTLE WITH THE HERB USED, THE EXTRACTION DATE, AND DOSAGE INSTRUCTIONS.

9. **<u>STORAGE AND USAGE</u>**: STORE THE TINCTURES IN A COOL, DARK PLACE AWAY FROM DIRECT SUNLIGHT OR HEAT. WHEN YOU WANT TO USE A TINCTURE, SHAKE THE BOTTLE WELL, AND USE THE RECOMMENDED DOSAGE AS PER YOUR NEEDS OR THE GUIDANCE OF A HEALTHCARE PROVIDER.

REMEMBER TO CONSULT WITH A HEALTHCARE PROFESSIONAL OR A QUALIFIED HERBALIST BEFORE USING HOMEMADE TINCTURES, ESPECIALLY IF YOU HAVE ANY UNDERLYING HEALTH CONDITIONS OR ARE TAKING MEDICATIONS.

WHEN PREPARING HERBAL TINCTURES AT HOME, IT'S IMPORTANT TO FOLLOW SAFETY GUIDELINES AND TAKE NECESSARY PRECAUTIONS. HERE ARE SOME KEY TIPS TO KEEP IN MIND:

1. **<u>CHOOSE SAFE HERBS</u>**: MAKE SURE YOU ARE USING HERBS THAT ARE SAFE FOR CONSUMPTION AND APPROPRIATE FOR TINCTURE PREPARATION. AVOID USING TOXIC OR POISONOUS PLANTS, AND ALWAYS RESEARCH THE SAFETY AND POTENTIAL INTERACTIONS OF EACH HERB BEFORE USE.

2. **<u>USE HIGH-QUALITY HERBS</u>**: OPT FOR ORGANIC, PESTICIDE-FREE, AND SUSTAINABLY SOURCED HERBS TO REDUCE THE RISK OF CONTAMINATION AND ENSURE THE POTENCY OF YOUR TINCTURE.

3. **<u>SANITIZE EQUIPMENT</u>**: BEFORE STARTING, MAKE SURE THAT ALL EQUIPMENT, INCLUDING THE GLASS JAR, MEASURING TOOLS, AND STRAINER, IS CLEAN AND SANITIZED. THIS HELPS PREVENT THE GROWTH OF BACTERIA OR MOLDS.

4. **<u>BE AWARE OF ALLERGIES</u>**: IF YOU HAVE KNOWN ALLERGIES TO SPECIFIC PLANTS OR HERBS, DO NOT USE

THEM IN YOUR TINCTURES. BE CAUTIOUS IF YOU ARE UNSURE ABOUT ANY POTENTIAL ALLERGIES OR SENSITIVITIES.

5. <u>SELECT AN APPROPRIATE ALCOHOL</u>: CHOOSE AN ALCOHOL WITH AT LEAST 40% ALCOHOL CONTENT, AS THIS HELPS EXTRACT THE MEDICINAL PROPERTIES FROM THE HERBS EFFECTIVELY. AVOID USING DENATURED ALCOHOL OR RUBBING ALCOHOL, AS THEY CONTAIN TOXIC ADDITIVES.

6. <u>AVOID CROSS-CONTAMINATION</u>: ENSURE THAT YOUR WORKSPACE IS CLEAN AND FREE FROM ANY CROSS-CONTAMINATION. USE SEPARATE UTENSILS AND EQUIPMENT FOR DIFFERENT HERBS TO AVOID MIXING SCENTS AND FLAVORS.

7. <u>LABEL AND STORE PROPERLY</u>: CLEARLY LABEL EACH BOTTLE OF TINCTURE WITH THE HERB USED, THE EXTRACTION DATE, AND DOSAGE INSTRUCTIONS. STORE THE TINCTURES IN DARK, COOL PLACES AWAY FROM DIRECT SUNLIGHT OR HEAT, AS EXPOSURE TO LIGHT AND HEAT CAN DEGRADE THE POTENCY OF THE TINCTURE.

8. **<u>CONSULT A PROFESSIONAL</u>**: IT'S ALWAYS A GOOD IDEA TO CONSULT WITH A HEALTHCARE PROFESSIONAL, HERBALIST, OR EXPERT BEFORE USING HOMEMADE TINCTURES, ESPECIALLY IF YOU HAVE UNDERLYING HEALTH CONDITIONS, ARE TAKING MEDICATIONS, OR IF YOU ARE PREGNANT OR BREASTFEEDING.

BY FOLLOWING THESE SAFETY GUIDELINES AND PRECAUTIONS, YOU CAN ENSURE THE QUALITY AND SAFETY OF YOUR HOMEMADE HERBAL TINCTURES.

CHAPTER 2

HERBAL TINCTURES CAN BE A GREAT WAY TO SUPPORT YOUR IMMUNE SYSTEM NATURALLY. HERE ARE A FEW HERBAL TINCTURE RECIPES THAT MAY HELP BOOST IMMUNITY:

1. **<u>ELDERBERRY TINCTURE</u>**:

- INGREDIENTS: 1 CUP DRIED ELDERBERRIES, 2 CUPS VODKA OR BRANDY

- INSTRUCTIONS: CRUSH THE DRIED ELDERBERRIES SLIGHTLY AND PLACE THEM IN A GLASS JAR. POUR THE VODKA OR BRANDY OVER THE ELDERBERRIES, ENSURING THEY ARE COMPLETELY COVERED. SEAL THE JAR TIGHTLY AND STORE IT IN A COOL, DARK PLACE FOR 4-6 WEEKS, SHAKING IT OCCASIONALLY. AFTER THE EXTRACTION PERIOD, STRAIN OUT THE ELDERBERRIES AND TRANSFER THE TINCTURE TO AMBER GLASS BOTTLES. TAKE 1 TEASPOON DAILY FOR IMMUNE SUPPORT.

2. **<u>ECHINACEA TINCTURE</u>**:

- INGREDIENTS: 1 CUP DRIED ECHINACEA ROOT, 2 CUPS VODKA OR BRANDY, 1 TABLESPOON GLYCERIN (OPTIONAL)

- INSTRUCTIONS: CHOP OR GRIND THE DRIED ECHINACEA ROOT AND PLACE IT IN A GLASS JAR. POUR THE VODKA OR BRANDY OVER THE ROOT, ENSURING IT IS FULLY IMMERSED. ADD GLYCERIN, IF DESIRED, TO ENHANCE SWEETNESS. SEAL

THE JAR TIGHTLY AND STORE IN A DARK PLACE FOR 4-6
WEEKS, SHAKING OCCASIONALLY. STRAIN OUT THE ROOT
AND TRANSFER THE TINCTURE TO AMBER GLASS BOTTLES.
TAKE 1 TEASPOON 3 TIMES A DAY DURING ILLNESS OR AS A
PREVENTIVE MEASURE.

3. **ASTRAGALUS TINCTURE**:

- INGREDIENTS: 1 CUP DRIED ASTRAGALUS ROOT SLICES, 2
CUPS VODKA OR BRANDY

- INSTRUCTIONS: PLACE THE DRIED ASTRAGALUS ROOT IN A
GLASS JAR AND POUR THE VODKA OR BRANDY OVER IT,
MAKING SURE THE ROOT IS COMPLETELY COVERED. SEAL
THE JAR TIGHTLY AND STORE IT IN A COOL, DARK PLACE FOR
6-8 WEEKS, SHAKING OCCASIONALLY. AFTER THE
EXTRACTION PERIOD, STRAIN THE ROOT AND TRANSFER THE
TINCTURE TO AMBER GLASS BOTTLES. TAKE 1 TEASPOON
DAILY TO SUPPORT THE IMMUNE SYSTEM.

REMEMBER TO CONSULT A HEALTHCARE PROFESSIONAL OR HERBALIST BEFORE USING ANY HERBAL TINCTURES, ESPECIALLY IF YOU HAVE ANY MEDICAL CONDITIONS OR ARE TAKING MEDICATIONS. THEY CAN ADVISE YOU ON THE APPROPRIATE DOSAGE AND DISCUSS ANY POTENTIAL INTERACTIONS WITH YOUR CURRENT HEALTH SITUATION.

HERBAL TINCTURES CAN BE A WONDERFUL NATURAL REMEDY FOR SUPPORTING DIGESTIVE HEALTH. BELOW ARE A FEW HERBAL TINCTURE RECIPES THAT MAY HELP ALLEVIATE COMMON DIGESTIVE ISSUES:

1. <u>**PEPPERMINT TINCTURE**</u>:

- INGREDIENTS: 1 CUP FRESH PEPPERMINT LEAVES, 2 CUPS VODKA OR BRANDY

- INSTRUCTIONS: CHOP OR CRUSH THE FRESH PEPPERMINT LEAVES AND PLACE THEM IN A GLASS JAR. POUR THE VODKA OR BRANDY OVER THE LEAVES, ENSURING THEY ARE FULLY COVERED. SEAL THE JAR TIGHTLY AND STORE IT IN A COOL, DARK PLACE FOR 4-6 WEEKS, SHAKING OCCASIONALLY. AFTER THE EXTRACTION PERIOD, STRAIN OUT THE LEAVES AND TRANSFER THE TINCTURE TO AMBER GLASS BOTTLES. TAKE 1 TEASPOON AS NEEDED FOR RELIEF FROM GAS, BLOATING, OR INDIGESTION.

2. **<u>GINGER TINCTURE</u>**:

- INGREDIENTS: 1 CUP FRESH GINGER ROOT, GRATED OR CHOPPED, 2 CUPS VODKA OR BRANDY

- INSTRUCTIONS: PLACE THE GRATED OR CHOPPED GINGER ROOT IN A GLASS JAR. POUR THE VODKA OR BRANDY OVER THE ROOT, ENSURING IT IS FULLY IMMERSED. SEAL THE JAR TIGHTLY AND STORE IT IN A COOL, DARK PLACE FOR 4-6 WEEKS, SHAKING OCCASIONALLY. STRAIN OUT THE ROOT AND TRANSFER THE TINCTURE TO AMBER GLASS BOTTLES. TAKE 1 TEASPOON BEFORE OR AFTER MEALS TO AID DIGESTION.

3. **<u>FENNEL TINCTURE</u>**:

- INGREDIENTS: 1 CUP DRIED FENNEL SEEDS, 2 CUPS VODKA OR BRANDY

- INSTRUCTIONS: CRUSH THE DRIED FENNEL SEEDS SLIGHTLY AND PLACE THEM IN A GLASS JAR. POUR THE VODKA OR BRANDY OVER THE SEEDS, ENSURING THEY ARE COMPLETELY COVERED. SEAL THE JAR TIGHTLY AND STORE IT IN A COOL, DARK PLACE FOR 6-8 WEEKS, SHAKING OCCASIONALLY. AFTER THE EXTRACTION PERIOD, STRAIN OUT THE SEEDS AND TRANSFER THE TINCTURE TO AMBER GLASS BOTTLES. TAKE 1 TEASPOON BEFORE MEALS TO HELP RELIEVE DIGESTIVE DISCOMFORT.

PLEASE NOTE THAT EVERYONE'S BODY IS UNIQUE, AND WHAT WORKS FOR ONE PERSON MAY NOT WORK FOR ANOTHER. IT'S CRUCIAL TO CONSULT A HEALTHCARE PROFESSIONAL OR A QUALIFIED HERBALIST BEFORE USING ANY HERBAL TINCTURES, ESPECIALLY IF YOU HAVE UNDERLYING HEALTH CONDITIONS, ARE PREGNANT OR BREASTFEEDING, OR ARE TAKING MEDICATIONS. THEY CAN GUIDE YOU ON THE PROPER DOSAGE AND USAGE FOR YOUR SPECIFIC NEEDS.

BELOW ARE A FEW HERBAL TINCTURE RECIPES THAT MAY HELP SUPPORT RESPIRATORY HEALTH:

1. <u>**ECHINACEA TINCTURE**</u>: (SEE PAGE 8)

2. <u>**MULLEIN LEAF TINCTURE**</u>:

- INGREDIENTS: 1 CUP DRIED MULLEIN LEAVES, 2 CUPS VODKA OR BRANDY

- INSTRUCTIONS: PLACE THE DRIED MULLEIN LEAVES IN A GLASS JAR. POUR THE VODKA OR BRANDY OVER THE LEAVES, ENSURING THEY ARE COMPLETELY COVERED. SEAL THE JAR TIGHTLY AND STORE IT IN A COOL, DARK PLACE FOR 4-6 WEEKS, SHAKING OCCASIONALLY. AFTER THE EXTRACTION PERIOD, STRAIN OUT THE LEAVES AND TRANSFER THE TINCTURE TO AMBER GLASS BOTTLES. TAKE 1 TEASPOON DAILY TO HELP SOOTHE RESPIRATORY ISSUES AND SUPPORT LUNG HEALTH.

3. <u>**THYME TINCTURE**</u>:

- INGREDIENTS: 1 CUP FRESH THYME LEAVES, 2 CUPS VODKA OR BRANDY

- INSTRUCTIONS: CHOP OR CRUSH THE FRESH THYME LEAVES AND PLACE THEM IN A GLASS JAR. POUR THE VODKA OR BRANDY OVER THE LEAVES, ENSURING THEY ARE FULLY COVERED. SEAL THE JAR TIGHTLY AND STORE IT IN A COOL,

DARK PLACE FOR 4-6 WEEKS, SHAKING OCCASIONALLY. STRAIN OUT THE LEAVES AND TRANSFER THE TINCTURE TO AMBER GLASS BOTTLES. TAKE 1 TEASPOON DAILY TO SUPPORT RESPIRATORY HEALTH AND RELIEVE CONGESTION.

AGAIN, IT'S IMPORTANT TO CONSULT WITH A HEALTHCARE PROFESSIONAL OR A QUALIFIED HERBALIST BEFORE USING ANY HERBAL TINCTURES, ESPECIALLY IF YOU HAVE UNDERLYING HEALTH CONDITIONS, ARE PREGNANT OR BREASTFEEDING, OR ARE TAKING MEDICATIONS. THEY CAN PROVIDE GUIDANCE ON THE PROPER DOSAGE AND USAGE FOR YOUR SPECIFIC NEEDS.

HERE ARE A FEW HERBAL TINCTURE RECIPES THAT MAY PROMOTE SLEEP AND RELAXATION:

1. **<u>VALERIAN ROOT TINCTURE</u>**:

- INGREDIENTS: 1 CUP DRIED VALERIAN ROOT, 2 CUPS VODKA OR BRANDY

- INSTRUCTIONS: PLACE THE DRIED VALERIAN ROOT IN A GLASS JAR. POUR THE VODKA OR BRANDY OVER THE ROOT, MAKING SURE IT IS FULLY COVERED. SEAL THE JAR TIGHTLY AND STORE IT IN A COOL, DARK PLACE FOR 4-6 WEEKS, SHAKING OCCASIONALLY. AFTER THE EXTRACTION PERIOD, STRAIN OUT THE ROOT AND TRANSFER THE TINCTURE TO AMBER GLASS BOTTLES. TAKE 1 TEASPOON BEFORE BEDTIME TO PROMOTE RELAXATION AND SUPPORT BETTER SLEEP.

2. **<u>CHAMOMILE TINCTURE</u>**:

- INGREDIENTS: 1 CUP DRIED CHAMOMILE FLOWERS, 2 CUPS VODKA OR BRANDY

- INSTRUCTIONS: PLACE THE DRIED CHAMOMILE FLOWERS IN A GLASS JAR. POUR THE VODKA OR BRANDY OVER THE FLOWERS, ENSURING THEY ARE COMPLETELY IMMERSED. SEAL THE JAR TIGHTLY AND STORE IT IN A COOL, DARK PLACE FOR 4-6 WEEKS, SHAKING OCCASIONALLY. STRAIN OUT THE FLOWERS AND TRANSFER THE TINCTURE TO AMBER

GLASS BOTTLES. TAKE 1 TEASPOON BEFORE BEDTIME TO HELP INDUCE RELAXATION AND IMPROVE SLEEP QUALITY.

3. **<u>PASSIONFLOWER TINCTURE</u>**:

- INGREDIENTS: 1 CUP DRIED PASSIONFLOWER LEAVES AND FLOWERS, 2 CUPS VODKA OR BRANDY

- INSTRUCTIONS: PLACE THE DRIED PASSIONFLOWER LEAVES AND FLOWERS IN A GLASS JAR. POUR THE VODKA OR BRANDY OVER THE HERB, ENSURING IT IS FULLY COVERED. SEAL THE JAR TIGHTLY AND STORE IT IN A COOL, DARK PLACE FOR 4-6 WEEKS, SHAKING OCCASIONALLY. AFTER THE EXTRACTION PERIOD, STRAIN OUT THE HERB AND TRANSFER THE TINCTURE TO AMBER GLASS BOTTLES. TAKE 1 TEASPOON BEFORE BEDTIME TO PROMOTE CALMNESS AND SUPPORT RESTFUL SLEEP.

AGAIN, IT'S ESSENTIAL TO CONSULT WITH A HEALTHCARE PROFESSIONAL OR A QUALIFIED HERBALIST BEFORE USING ANY HERBAL TINCTURES, ESPECIALLY IF YOU HAVE UNDERLYING HEALTH CONDITIONS, ARE PREGNANT OR BREASTFEEDING, OR ARE TAKING MEDICATIONS. THEY CAN PROVIDE GUIDANCE ON THE PROPER DOSAGE AND USAGE FOR YOUR SPECIFIC NEEDS.

HERE ARE A FEW HERBAL TINCTURE RECIPES THAT MAY HELP BOOST ENERGY AND VITALITY:

1. **ELEUTHERO ROOT TINCTURE**:

- INGREDIENTS: 1 CUP DRIED ELEUTHERO ROOT, 2 CUPS VODKA OR BRANDY

- INSTRUCTIONS: PLACE THE DRIED ELEUTHERO ROOT IN A GLASS JAR. POUR THE VODKA OR BRANDY OVER THE ROOT, ENSURING IT IS FULLY COVERED. SEAL THE JAR TIGHTLY AND STORE IT IN A COOL, DARK PLACE FOR 4-6 WEEKS, SHAKING OCCASIONALLY. AFTER THE EXTRACTION PERIOD, STRAIN OUT THE ROOT AND TRANSFER THE TINCTURE TO AMBER GLASS BOTTLES. TAKE 1 TEASPOON IN THE MORNING TO SUPPORT ENERGY AND VITALITY.

2. **GINSENG TINCTURE**:

- INGREDIENTS: 1 CUP DRIED GINSENG ROOT, 2 CUPS VODKA OR BRANDY

- INSTRUCTIONS: PLACE THE DRIED GINSENG ROOT IN A GLASS JAR. POUR THE VODKA OR BRANDY OVER THE ROOT, MAKING SURE IT IS FULLY COVERED. SEAL THE JAR TIGHTLY AND STORE IT IN A COOL, DARK PLACE FOR 4-6 WEEKS, SHAKING OCCASIONALLY. STRAIN OUT THE ROOT AND TRANSFER THE TINCTURE TO AMBER GLASS BOTTLES. TAKE 1

TEASPOON IN THE MORNING TO HELP INCREASE ENERGY AND PROMOTE OVERALL VITALITY.

3. <u>**MACA ROOT TINCTURE**</u>:

- INGREDIENTS: 1 CUP DRIED MACA ROOT, 2 CUPS VODKA OR BRANDY

- INSTRUCTIONS: PLACE THE DRIED MACA ROOT IN A GLASS JAR. POUR THE VODKA OR BRANDY OVER THE ROOT, ENSURING IT IS FULLY COVERED. SEAL THE JAR TIGHTLY AND STORE IT IN A COOL, DARK PLACE FOR 4-6 WEEKS, SHAKING OCCASIONALLY. AFTER THE EXTRACTION PERIOD, STRAIN OUT THE ROOT AND TRANSFER THE TINCTURE TO AMBER GLASS BOTTLES. TAKE 1 TEASPOON IN THE MORNING TO SUPPORT ENERGY LEVELS AND ENHANCE VITALITY.

REMEMBER TO CONSULT WITH A HEALTHCARE PROFESSIONAL OR A QUALIFIED HERBALIST BEFORE USING ANY HERBAL TINCTURES, ESPECIALLY IF YOU HAVE UNDERLYING HEALTH CONDITIONS, ARE PREGNANT OR BREASTFEEDING, OR ARE TAKING MEDICATIONS. THEY CAN PROVIDE GUIDANCE ON THE PROPER DOSAGE AND USAGE FOR YOUR SPECIFIC NEEDS.

HERE ARE A FEW HERBAL TINCTURE RECIPES THAT MAY HELP WITH MUSCLE AND JOINT AILMENTS:

1. <u>**ARNICA TINCTURE**</u>:

- INGREDIENTS: 1 CUP DRIED ARNICA FLOWERS, 2 CUPS RUBBING ALCOHOL OR HIGH-PROOF VODKA

- INSTRUCTIONS: PLACE THE DRIED ARNICA FLOWERS IN A GLASS JAR. POUR THE RUBBING ALCOHOL OR VODKA OVER THE FLOWERS, ENSURING THEY ARE FULLY COVERED. SEAL THE JAR TIGHTLY AND STORE IT IN A COOL, DARK PLACE FOR 4-6 WEEKS, SHAKING OCCASIONALLY. AFTER THE EXTRACTION PERIOD, STRAIN OUT THE FLOWERS AND TRANSFER THE TINCTURE TO AMBER GLASS BOTTLES. APPLY TOPICALLY TO SORE MUSCLES AND JOINTS AS NEEDED. AVOID APPLYING TO BROKEN SKIN.

2. **<u>TURMERIC TINCTURE</u>**:

- INGREDIENTS: 1 CUP CHOPPED FRESH TURMERIC ROOT OR 1/2 CUP DRIED TURMERIC ROOT POWDER, 2 CUPS VODKA OR BRANDY

- INSTRUCTIONS: PLACE THE FRESH TURMERIC ROOT OR TURMERIC POWDER IN A GLASS JAR. POUR THE VODKA OR BRANDY OVER IT, MAKING SURE IT IS FULLY COVERED. SEAL THE JAR TIGHTLY AND STORE IT IN A COOL, DARK PLACE FOR 4-6 WEEKS, SHAKING OCCASIONALLY. AFTER THE EXTRACTION PERIOD, STRAIN OUT THE TURMERIC AND TRANSFER THE TINCTURE TO AMBER GLASS BOTTLES. TAKE 1 TEASPOON ORALLY TWICE A DAY TO SUPPORT JOINT HEALTH AND REDUCE INFLAMMATION.

3. **<u>STINGING NETTLE TINCTURE</u>**:

- INGREDIENTS: 1 CUP DRIED STINGING NETTLE LEAVES, 2 CUPS VODKA OR BRANDY

- INSTRUCTIONS: PLACE THE DRIED STINGING NETTLE LEAVES IN A GLASS JAR. POUR THE VODKA OR BRANDY OVER THE LEAVES, ENSURING THEY ARE FULLY COVERED. SEAL THE JAR TIGHTLY AND STORE IT IN A COOL, DARK PLACE FOR 4-6 WEEKS, SHAKING OCCASIONALLY. AFTER THE EXTRACTION PERIOD, STRAIN OUT THE LEAVES AND TRANSFER THE TINCTURE TO AMBER GLASS BOTTLES. TAKE 1

TEASPOON ORALLY TWICE A DAY TO ALLEVIATE JOINT PAIN AND INFLAMMATION.

HERE ARE A FEW HERBAL TINCTURE RECIPES THAT MAY HELP WITH STRESS AND ANXIETY:

1. <u>**LEMON BALM TINCTURE**</u>:

- INGREDIENTS: 1 CUP DRIED LEMON BALM LEAVES, 2 CUPS VODKA OR BRANDY

- INSTRUCTIONS: PLACE THE DRIED LEMON BALM LEAVES IN A GLASS JAR. POUR THE VODKA OR BRANDY OVER THE LEAVES, ENSURING THEY ARE FULLY COVERED. SEAL THE JAR TIGHTLY AND STORE IT IN A COOL, DARK PLACE FOR 4-6 WEEKS, SHAKING OCCASIONALLY. AFTER THE EXTRACTION PERIOD, STRAIN OUT THE LEAVES AND TRANSFER THE TINCTURE TO AMBER GLASS BOTTLES. TAKE 1 TEASPOON ORALLY THREE TIMES A DAY TO PROMOTE RELAXATION AND REDUCE STRESS.

2. <u>**CHAMOMILE TINCTURE**</u>: (SEE PAGE 11)

3. <u>**PASSIONFLOWER TINCTURE**</u>: (SEE PAGE 11)

AGAIN, IT IS IMPORTANT TO CONSULT WITH A HEALTHCARE PROFESSIONAL OR A QUALIFIED HERBALIST BEFORE USING ANY HERBAL TINCTURES, ESPECIALLY IF YOU HAVE UNDERLYING HEALTH CONDITIONS, ARE PREGNANT OR BREASTFEEDING, OR ARE TAKING MEDICATIONS. THEY CAN PROVIDE GUIDANCE ON THE PROPER USAGE AND DOSAGE FOR YOUR SPECIFIC NEEDS.

CHAPTER 3

HEAD AND SINUSES

HERE ARE A FEW HERBAL TINCTURE RECIPES THAT MAY HELP WITH HEAD AND SINUS ISSUES:

1. **<u>EUCALYPTUS TINCTURE</u>**:

- INGREDIENTS: 1 CUP DRIED EUCALYPTUS LEAVES, 2 CUPS VODKA OR BRANDY

- INSTRUCTIONS: PLACE THE DRIED EUCALYPTUS LEAVES IN A GLASS JAR. POUR THE VODKA OR BRANDY OVER THE LEAVES, ENSURING THEY ARE FULLY COVERED. SEAL THE JAR TIGHTLY AND STORE IT IN A COOL, DARK PLACE FOR 4-6 WEEKS, SHAKING OCCASIONALLY. AFTER THE EXTRACTION PERIOD, STRAIN OUT THE LEAVES AND TRANSFER THE TINCTURE TO AMBER GLASS BOTTLES. TAKE 1 TEASPOON ORALLY THREE TIMES A DAY TO EASE SINUS CONGESTION AND PROMOTE CLEAR BREATHING.

2. **<u>PEPPERMINT TINCTURE</u>**: (SEE PAGE 9)

3. **<u>YARROW TINCTURE</u>**:

- INGREDIENTS: 1 CUP DRIED YARROW FLOWERS AND LEAVES, 2 CUPS VODKA OR BRANDY

- INSTRUCTIONS: PLACE THE DRIED YARROW FLOWERS AND LEAVES IN A GLASS JAR. POUR THE VODKA OR BRANDY OVER THEM, ENSURING THEY ARE FULLY COVERED. SEAL THE JAR TIGHTLY AND STORE IT IN A COOL, DARK PLACE FOR 4-6 WEEKS, SHAKING OCCASIONALLY. AFTER THE EXTRACTION PERIOD, STRAIN OUT THE FLOWERS AND LEAVES AND TRANSFER THE TINCTURE TO AMBER GLASS BOTTLES. TAKE 1 TEASPOON ORALLY THREE TIMES A DAY TO REDUCE INFLAMMATION AND EASE SINUS PRESSURE.

AS ALWAYS, IT IS ADVISABLE TO CONSULT WITH A HEALTHCARE PROFESSIONAL OR A QUALIFIED HERBALIST BEFORE USING ANY HERBAL TINCTURES, ESPECIALLY IF YOU HAVE UNDERLYING HEALTH CONDITIONS, ARE PREGNANT OR BREASTFEEDING, OR ARE TAKING MEDICATIONS. THEY CAN PROVIDE GUIDANCE ON THE PROPER USAGE AND DOSAGE FOR YOUR SPECIFIC NEEDS.

HERE ARE A FEW HERBAL TINCTURE RECIPES THAT MAY HELP WITH THROAT AND RESPIRATORY AILMENTS:

1. <u>**SAGE TINCTURE**</u>:

- INGREDIENTS: 1 CUP DRIED SAGE LEAVES, 2 CUPS VODKA OR BRANDY

- INSTRUCTIONS: PLACE THE DRIED SAGE LEAVES IN A GLASS JAR. POUR THE VODKA OR BRANDY OVER THE LEAVES, ENSURING THEY ARE FULLY COVERED. SEAL THE JAR TIGHTLY AND STORE IT IN A COOL, DARK PLACE FOR 4-6 WEEKS, SHAKING OCCASIONALLY. AFTER THE EXTRACTION PERIOD, STRAIN OUT THE LEAVES AND TRANSFER THE TINCTURE TO AMBER GLASS BOTTLES. TAKE 1 TEASPOON ORALLY THREE TIMES A DAY TO SOOTHE SORE THROAT AND REDUCE INFLAMMATION IN THE RESPIRATORY SYSTEM.

2. <u>**MARSHMALLOW ROOT TINCTURE**</u>:

- INGREDIENTS: 1 CUP DRIED MARSHMALLOW ROOT, 2 CUPS VODKA OR BRANDY

- INSTRUCTIONS: PLACE THE DRIED MARSHMALLOW ROOT IN A GLASS JAR. POUR THE VODKA OR BRANDY OVER THE ROOT, ENSURING IT IS FULLY COVERED. SEAL THE JAR TIGHTLY AND STORE IT IN A COOL, DARK PLACE FOR 4-6 WEEKS, SHAKING

OCCASIONALLY. AFTER THE EXTRACTION PERIOD, STRAIN OUT THE ROOT AND TRANSFER THE TINCTURE TO AMBER GLASS BOTTLES. TAKE 1 TEASPOON ORALLY THREE TIMES A DAY TO RELIEVE SORE THROAT, COUGH, AND RESPIRATORY CONGESTION.

3. **<u>MULLEIN TINCTURE</u>**:

- INGREDIENTS: 1 CUP DRIED MULLEIN LEAVES AND FLOWERS, 2 CUPS VODKA OR BRANDY

- INSTRUCTIONS: PLACE THE DRIED MULLEIN LEAVES AND FLOWERS IN A GLASS JAR. POUR THE VODKA OR BRANDY OVER THEM, ENSURING THEY ARE FULLY COVERED. SEAL THE JAR TIGHTLY AND STORE IT IN A COOL, DARK PLACE FOR 4-6 WEEKS, SHAKING OCCASIONALLY. AFTER THE EXTRACTION PERIOD, STRAIN OUT THE LEAVES AND FLOWERS AND TRANSFER THE TINCTURE TO AMBER GLASS BOTTLES. TAKE 1 TEASPOON ORALLY THREE TIMES A DAY TO RELIEVE RESPIRATORY CONGESTION, SOOTHE A SORE THROAT, AND REDUCE COUGH.

AGAIN, IT'S IMPORTANT TO CONSULT WITH A HEALTHCARE PROFESSIONAL OR HERBALIST BEFORE USING HERBAL TINCTURES, ESPECIALLY IF YOU HAVE ANY UNDERLYING HEALTH CONDITIONS, ARE PREGNANT OR

BREASTFEEDING, OR ARE TAKING MEDICATIONS. THEY CAN PROVIDE GUIDANCE ON THE PROPER USAGE AND DOSAGE FOR YOUR SPECIFIC NEEDS.

<u>*DIGESTIVE SYSTEM*</u>

HERE ARE A FEW HERBAL TINCTURE RECIPES THAT MAY HELP SUPPORT THE DIGESTIVE SYSTEM:

1. **<u>PEPPERMINT TINCTURE</u>**: (SEE PAGE 9)

2. **<u>GINGER TINCTURE</u>**: (SEE PAGE 9)

3. **<u>DANDELION ROOT TINCTURE</u>**:

- INGREDIENTS: 1 CUP DRIED DANDELION ROOTS, 2 CUPS VODKA OR BRANDY

- INSTRUCTIONS: PLACE THE DRIED DANDELION ROOTS IN A GLASS JAR. POUR THE VODKA OR BRANDY OVER THE ROOTS, ENSURING THEY ARE FULLY COVERED. SEAL THE JAR TIGHTLY AND STORE IT IN A COOL, DARK PLACE FOR 4-6 WEEKS, SHAKING OCCASIONALLY. AFTER THE EXTRACTION PERIOD, STRAIN OUT THE ROOTS AND TRANSFER THE TINCTURE TO AMBER GLASS BOTTLES. TAKE 1 TEASPOON ORALLY THREE TIMES A DAY TO SUPPORT LIVER FUNCTION, STIMULATE BILE PRODUCTION, AND AID DIGESTION.

AGAIN, IT IS IMPORTANT TO CONSULT WITH A HEALTHCARE PROFESSIONAL OR HERBALIST BEFORE USING HERBAL TINCTURES, ESPECIALLY IF YOU HAVE ANY UNDERLYING HEALTH CONDITIONS, ARE PREGNANT OR BREASTFEEDING, OR ARE TAKING MEDICATIONS. THEY CAN PROVIDE GUIDANCE APPROPRIATE FOR YOUR SPECIFIC NEEDS.

HERE ARE A FEW HERBAL TINCTURE RECIPES THAT MAY HELP SUPPORT MUSCLES AND JOINTS:

1. **<u>ARNICA TINCTURE</u>**: (SEE PAGE 13)

2. **<u>TURMERIC TINCTURE</u>**: (SEE PAGE 13)

3. **<u>COMFREY TINCTURE</u>**:

- INGREDIENTS: 1 CUP DRIED COMFREY LEAVES, 2 CUPS VODKA OR BRANDY

- INSTRUCTIONS: PLACE THE DRIED COMFREY LEAVES IN A GLASS JAR. POUR THE VODKA OR BRANDY OVER THE LEAVES, ENSURING THEY ARE FULLY COVERED. SEAL THE JAR TIGHTLY AND STORE IT IN A COOL, DARK PLACE FOR 4-6 WEEKS, SHAKING OCCASIONALLY. AFTER THE EXTRACTION PERIOD, STRAIN OUT THE LEAVES AND TRANSFER THE TINCTURE TO AMBER GLASS BOTTLES. APPLY TOPICALLY TO PROMOTE HEALING OF SPRAINS, STRAINS, AND MINOR WOUNDS. DO NOT USE ON BROKEN SKIN OR FOR LONG PERIODS WITHOUT CONSULTING A HEALTHCARE PROFESSIONAL.

AS ALWAYS, IT IS IMPORTANT TO CONSULT WITH A HEALTHCARE PROFESSIONAL OR HERBALIST BEFORE USING HERBAL TINCTURES, ESPECIALLY IF YOU HAVE ANY UNDERLYING HEALTH CONDITIONS OR ARE TAKING MEDICATIONS. THEY CAN PROVIDE GUIDANCE APPROPRIATE FOR YOUR SPECIFIC NEEDS.

HERE ARE A FEW HERBAL TINCTURE RECIPES THAT MAY BENEFIT THE SKIN AND HAIR:

1. **CALENDULA TINCTURE**:

- INGREDIENTS: 1 CUP DRIED CALENDULA FLOWERS, 2 CUPS VODKA OR BRANDY

- INSTRUCTIONS: PLACE THE DRIED CALENDULA FLOWERS IN A GLASS JAR. POUR THE VODKA OR BRANDY OVER THE FLOWERS, ENSURING THEY ARE FULLY COVERED. SEAL THE JAR TIGHTLY AND STORE IT IN A COOL, DARK PLACE FOR 4-6 WEEKS, SHAKING OCCASIONALLY. AFTER THE EXTRACTION PERIOD, STRAIN OUT THE FLOWERS AND TRANSFER THE TINCTURE TO AMBER GLASS BOTTLES. APPLY TOPICALLY TO SOOTHE AND HEAL VARIOUS SKIN CONDITIONS SUCH AS INFLAMMATION, IRRITATION, AND WOUNDS.

2. <u>**ROSEMARY TINCTURE**</u>:

- INGREDIENTS: 1 CUP FRESH ROSEMARY LEAVES, 2 CUPS VODKA OR BRANDY

- INSTRUCTIONS: PLACE THE FRESH ROSEMARY LEAVES IN A GLASS JAR. POUR THE VODKA OR BRANDY OVER THE LEAVES, ENSURING THEY ARE FULLY COVERED. SEAL THE JAR TIGHTLY AND STORE IT IN A COOL, DARK PLACE FOR 4-6 WEEKS, SHAKING OCCASIONALLY. AFTER THE EXTRACTION PERIOD, STRAIN OUT THE LEAVES AND TRANSFER THE TINCTURE TO AMBER GLASS BOTTLES. APPLY TOPICALLY TO STIMULATE HAIR GROWTH, STRENGTHEN HAIR FOLLICLES, AND ENHANCE SCALP HEALTH. IT CAN ALSO BE ADDED TO HOMEMADE HAIR CARE PRODUCTS.

3. <u>**CHAMOMILE TINCTURE**</u>: (SEE PAGE 11)

ALWAYS PERFORM A PATCH TEST BEFORE USING HERBAL TINCTURES DIRECTLY ON YOUR SKIN OR SCALP, AS SOME INDIVIDUALS MAY HAVE SENSITIVITIES OR ALLERGIES TO CERTAIN HERBS. IF ANY ADVERSE REACTIONS OCCUR, DISCONTINUE USE IMMEDIATELY. IT IS ALSO ADVISABLE TO CONSULT WITH A HEALTHCARE PROFESSIONAL OR HERBALIST TO ENSURE THE APPROPRIATE USE AND DOSAGE FOR YOUR SPECIFIC NEEDS.

CHAPTER 4

RECIPES FOR SPECIFIC AILMENTS AND BODY SECTIONS

4.1 <u>IMMUNE SYSTEM SUPPORT</u>

ELDERBERRY ELIXIR IS WIDELY USED AS A NATURAL REMEDY TO SUPPORT THE IMMUNE SYSTEM AND ALLEVIATE SYMPTOMS OF THE COLD AND FLU. HERE'S A SIMPLE RECIPE TO MAKE YOUR OWN ELDERBERRY ELIXIR:

<u>INGREDIENTS:</u>

- 1 CUP DRIED ELDERBERRIES

- 4 CUPS WATER

- 1 CUP RAW HONEY

- OPTIONAL: ADDITIONAL HERBS SUCH AS GINGER OR CINNAMON FOR ADDED IMMUNE SUPPORT

<u>INSTRUCTIONS:</u>

1. IN A MEDIUM-SIZED SAUCEPAN, COMBINE THE DRIED ELDERBERRIES AND WATER.

2. BRING THE MIXTURE TO A BOIL, THEN REDUCE THE HEAT TO LOW AND LET IT SIMMER FOR ABOUT 30-45 MINUTES UNTIL THE LIQUID HAS REDUCED BY HALF.

3. REMOVE THE SAUCEPAN FROM THE HEAT AND ALLOW THE MIXTURE TO COOL SLIGHTLY.

4. USE A FINE MESH STRAINER OR CHEESECLOTH TO STRAIN OUT THE ELDERBERRIES, PRESSING ON THEM TO EXTRACT AS MUCH LIQUID AS POSSIBLE.

5. LET THE LIQUID COOL COMPLETELY BEFORE ADDING THE RAW HONEY.

6. STIR THE HONEY INTO THE ELDERBERRY LIQUID UNTIL IT DISSOLVES COMPLETELY.

7. IF DESIRED, YOU CAN ADD ADDITIONAL IMMUNE-SUPPORTING HERBS, SUCH AS GRATED FRESH GINGER OR A CINNAMON STICK. SIMMER THESE ADDED HERBS IN THE LIQUID FOR ANOTHER 10 MINUTES BEFORE STRAINING THEM OUT.

8. POUR THE ELDERBERRY ELIXIR INTO A STERILIZED GLASS BOTTLE OR JAR FOR STORAGE. IT CAN BE STORED IN THE REFRIGERATOR FOR UP TO A MONTH.

TO USE, TAKE 1-2 TABLESPOONS OF ELDERBERRY ELIXIR
EVERY FEW HOURS AT THE ONSET OF COLD OR FLU
SYMPTOMS. YOU CAN ALSO TAKE IT AS A DAILY IMMUNE
BOOSTER DURING FLU SEASON OR WHEN YOU FEEL YOUR
IMMUNITY MAY BE COMPROMISED.

*NOTE: WHILE ELDERBERRY HAS BEEN TRADITIONALLY
USED FOR ITS IMMUNE-SUPPORTING PROPERTIES, IT'S
IMPORTANT TO CONSULT WITH A HEALTHCARE
PROFESSIONAL OR HERBALIST, ESPECIALLY IF YOU ARE ON
MEDICATION OR HAVE ANY UNDERLYING HEALTH
CONDITIONS.*

ECHINACEA AND GOLDENSEAL BLEND FOR IMMUNE BOOST

ECHINACEA AND GOLDENSEAL ARE TWO HERBS
COMMONLY USED TOGETHER TO ENHANCE IMMUNE
FUNCTION AND BOOST OVERALL WELLNESS. HERE'S A BLEND
RECIPE TO MAKE YOUR OWN IMMUNE-BOOSTING ECHINACEA
AND GOLDENSEAL BLEND:

INGREDIENTS:

- 1/4 CUP DRIED ECHINACEA ROOT

- 1/4 CUP DRIED GOLDENSEAL ROOT

- OPTIONAL: ADDITIONAL IMMUNE-SUPPORTING HERBS LIKE ASTRAGALUS OR ELDERBERRY

INSTRUCTIONS:

1. IN A BOWL, COMBINE THE DRIED ECHINACEA ROOT AND DRIED GOLDENSEAL ROOT.

2. ADD ANY ADDITIONAL IMMUNE-SUPPORTING HERBS, IF DESIRED.

3. STIR THE HERBS TOGETHER UNTIL WELL COMBINED.

4. STORE THE BLEND IN AN AIRTIGHT CONTAINER, AWAY FROM DIRECT SUNLIGHT AND MOISTURE.

TO USE, FOLLOW THESE GUIDELINES:

- FOR PREVENTION AND GENERAL IMMUNE SUPPORT: TAKE 1 TEASPOON OF THE BLEND DAILY. YOU CAN MIX IT WITH A LITTLE WATER OR ADD IT TO YOUR FAVORITE HERBAL TEA.

- WHEN FEELING UNDER THE WEATHER OR AT THE ONSET OF COLD OR FLU SYMPTOMS: TAKE 1 TEASPOON OF THE BLEND

EVERY 2-3 HOURS, UP TO 8 TIMES PER DAY, FOR A MAXIMUM OF ONE WEEK.

- CONSULT A HEALTHCARE PROFESSIONAL OR HERBALIST IF YOU HAVE ANY UNDERLYING HEALTH CONDITIONS, ARE ON MEDICATION, OR IF YOU ARE PREGNANT OR BREASTFEEDING.

NOTE: ECHINACEA AND GOLDENSEAL ARE GENERALLY SAFE FOR SHORT-TERM USE, BUT IT'S BEST TO USE THEM UNDER THE GUIDANCE OF A HEALTHCARE PROFESSIONAL. THEY MAY INTERACT WITH CERTAIN MEDICATIONS OR HAVE CONTRAINDICATIONS FOR CERTAIN INDIVIDUALS.

4.2 **DIGESTIVE HEALTH**

PEPPERMINT AND GINGER ARE TWO HERBS KNOWN FOR THEIR DIGESTIVE BENEFITS. COMBINING THEM CREATES A POWERFUL TONIC TO SUPPORT DIGESTION AND ALLEVIATE VARIOUS DIGESTIVE ISSUES. HERE'S A SIMPLE RECIPE TO MAKE YOUR OWN PEPPERMINT AND GINGER DIGESTIVE TONIC:

INGREDIENTS:

- 1-INCH PIECE OF FRESH GINGER ROOT, GRATED

- 1 TABLESPOON DRIED PEPPERMINT LEAVES (OR 3 TABLESPOONS FRESH PEPPERMINT LEAVES)

- 2 CUPS WATER

- OPTIONAL: HONEY OR LEMON FOR TASTE

INSTRUCTIONS:

1. IN A SMALL POT, ADD THE GRATED GINGER ROOT AND DRIED PEPPERMINT LEAVES.

2. POUR WATER OVER THE HERBS AND BRING THE MIXTURE TO A BOIL.

3. REDUCE HEAT AND LET IT SIMMER FOR ABOUT 10 MINUTES.

4. REMOVE THE POT FROM HEAT AND LET IT COOL FOR A FEW MINUTES.

5. STRAIN THE LIQUID INTO A MUG OR GLASS BOTTLE, DISCARDING THE GINGER AND LEAVES.

6. IF DESIRED, ADD HONEY OR LEMON FOR TASTE.

7. DRINK THE TONIC WARM OR CHILL IT IN THE REFRIGERATOR BEFORE CONSUMING.

<u>TO USE, FOLLOW THESE GUIDELINES:</u>

- FOR GENERAL DIGESTIVE SUPPORT OR TO SOOTHE AN UPSET STOMACH: DRINK 1 CUP OF THE TONIC AFTER MEALS OR AS NEEDED.

- TO RELIEVE BLOATING OR DIGESTIVE DISCOMFORT: SIP ON THE TONIC THROUGHOUT THE DAY OR AS NEEDED.

- CONSULT A HEALTHCARE PROFESSIONAL IF YOU HAVE SEVERE DIGESTIVE ISSUES OR GASTROINTESTINAL DISORDERS.

NOTE: GINGER AND PEPPERMINT ARE GENERALLY SAFE FOR MOST PEOPLE, BUT IT'S RECOMMENDED TO USE THEM IN MODERATION. IF YOU HAVE ANY UNDERLYING HEALTH CONDITIONS, ARE ON MEDICATION, OR IF YOU ARE PREGNANT OR BREASTFEEDING, CONSULT A HEALTHCARE PROFESSIONAL BEFORE USING THIS TONIC.

DANDELION AND BURDOCK ARE TWO POWERFUL HERBS THAT HAVE BEEN TRADITIONALLY USED TO SUPPORT HEALTHY DIGESTION. MAKING YOUR OWN DANDELION AND BURDOCK BITTERS IS A GREAT WAY TO INCORPORATE THESE HERBS INTO YOUR ROUTINE. HERE'S A RECIPE TO MAKE YOUR OWN DIGESTIVE BITTERS:

INGREDIENTS:

- 1 CUP DRIED DANDELION ROOT

- 1 CUP DRIED BURDOCK ROOT

- 2 CUPS HIGH-PROOF ALCOHOL (SUCH AS VODKA OR BRANDY)

- OPTIONAL: HONEY OR MAPLE SYRUP FOR TASTE

INSTRUCTIONS:

1. IN A GLASS JAR OR BOTTLE, COMBINE THE DRIED DANDELION ROOT AND BURDOCK ROOT.

2. POUR THE HIGH-PROOF ALCOHOL OVER THE HERBS, MAKING SURE THEY ARE FULLY SUBMERGED.

3. SEAL THE JAR OR BOTTLE TIGHTLY AND STORE IT IN A COOL, DARK PLACE FOR ABOUT 4-6 WEEKS. SHAKE THE JAR EVERY FEW DAYS TO AGITATE THE MIXTURE.

4. AFTER THE STEEPING PERIOD, STRAIN THE LIQUID INTO A CLEAN GLASS BOTTLE, DISCARDING THE HERBS.

5. IF DESIRED, ADD HONEY OR MAPLE SYRUP TO SWEETEN THE TASTE. START WITH A SMALL AMOUNT AND ADJUST TO YOUR PREFERENCE.

6. TIGHTLY SEAL THE BOTTLE AND STORE IT IN A COOL, DARK PLACE UNTIL READY TO USE.

TO USE THE DIGESTIVE BITTERS:

- TAKE 1 TEASPOON TO 1 TABLESPOON OF THE BITTERS BEFORE OR AFTER MEALS, DEPENDING ON YOUR PREFERENCE.

- YOU CAN TAKE THE BITTERS DIRECTLY ON THE TONGUE OR DILUTE THEM IN A SMALL AMOUNT OF WATER.

- BITTERS ARE BEST ENJOYED IN SMALL SIPS, ALLOWING THE TASTE TO LINGER IN YOUR MOUTH, WHICH ALSO HELPS STIMULATE DIGESTIVE ENZYMES.

NOTE: DANDELION AND BURDOCK BITTERS SHOULD BE USED IN MODERATION. IF YOU HAVE ANY UNDERLYING HEALTH CONDITIONS, ARE ON MEDICATION, OR IF YOU ARE PREGNANT OR BREASTFEEDING, CONSULT A HEALTHCARE PROFESSIONAL BEFORE USING THIS TONIC. ADDITIONALLY, IF YOU EXPERIENCE ANY ADVERSE REACTIONS, DISCONTINUE USE AND SEEK MEDICAL ADVICE.

4.3 <u>RESPIRATORY HEALTH</u>

MULLEIN AND MARSHMALLOW ROOT ARE BOTH SOOTHING HERBS THAT CAN HELP PROVIDE RELIEF FOR COUGHS AND THROAT IRRITATIONS. MAKING A SYRUP WITH THESE HERBS IS A GREAT WAY TO HARNESS THEIR BENEFITS. HERE'S A RECIPE TO MAKE YOUR OWN MULLEIN AND MARSHMALLOW ROOT SYRUP:

<u>INGREDIENTS:</u>

- 1/4 CUP DRIED MULLEIN LEAVES

- 1/4 CUP DRIED MARSHMALLOW ROOT

- 3 CUPS WATER

- 1 CUP HONEY

<u>INSTRUCTIONS:</u>

1. IN A MEDIUM-SIZED SAUCEPAN, COMBINE THE DRIED MULLEIN LEAVES, DRIED MARSHMALLOW ROOT, AND WATER.

2. BRING THE MIXTURE TO A BOIL, THEN REDUCE THE HEAT TO LOW AND LET IT SIMMER FOR ABOUT 30 MINUTES, OR UNTIL THE LIQUID HAS SIGNIFICANTLY REDUCED.

3. REMOVE THE MIXTURE FROM THE HEAT AND LET IT COOL FOR A FEW MINUTES.

4. STRAIN THE LIQUID INTO A CLEAN JAR OR BOWL, PRESSING ON THE HERBS TO EXTRACT AS MUCH LIQUID AS POSSIBLE.

5. DISCARD THE HERBS AND RETURN THE LIQUID TO THE SAUCEPAN.

6. OVER LOW HEAT, SLOWLY ADD THE HONEY TO THE LIQUID, STIRRING CONSTANTLY UNTIL WELL COMBINED.

7. ONCE THE HONEY IS COMPLETELY MIXED IN, REMOVE THE SYRUP FROM HEAT AND LET IT COOL.

8. TRANSFER THE SYRUP INTO A CLEAN, AIRTIGHT JAR AND STORE IT IN THE REFRIGERATOR.

<u>TO USE THE COUGH SYRUP:</u>

- TAKE 1 TEASPOON TO 1 TABLESPOON OF THE SYRUP AS NEEDED FOR COUGH RELIEF.

- THE SYRUP CAN BE TAKEN DIRECTLY FROM THE SPOON OR MIXED INTO A HOT DRINK LIKE HERBAL TEA FOR ADDED COMFORT.

NOTE: WHILE MULLEIN AND MARSHMALLOW ROOT ARE GENERALLY SAFE FOR MOST PEOPLE, IT'S ALWAYS A GOOD IDEA TO CONSULT A HEALTHCARE PROFESSIONAL BEFORE USING THEM, ESPECIALLY IF YOU HAVE ANY UNDERLYING HEALTH CONDITIONS, ARE ON MEDICATION, OR IF YOU ARE PREGNANT OR BREASTFEEDING. ADDITIONALLY, IF YOUR COUGH PERSISTS OR WORSENS, SEEK MEDICAL ADVICE.

THYME AND EUCALYPTUS ARE BOTH POWERFUL HERBS THAT HAVE BEEN TRADITIONALLY USED TO SUPPORT RESPIRATORY HEALTH AND ALLEVIATE CONGESTION. MAKING A RESPIRATORY TONIC WITH THESE HERBS CAN HELP PROVIDE RELIEF AND PROMOTE A HEALTHY RESPIRATORY SYSTEM. HERE'S A RECIPE TO MAKE YOUR OWN THYME AND EUCALYPTUS RESPIRATORY TONIC:

INGREDIENTS:

- 1 TABLESPOON DRIED THYME LEAVES

- 1 TABLESPOON DRIED EUCALYPTUS LEAVES

- 2 CUPS WATER

- 1 TABLESPOON HONEY (OPTIONAL)

- LEMON JUICE (OPTIONAL)

<u>**INSTRUCTIONS:**</u>

1. IN A SMALL SAUCEPAN, COMBINE THE DRIED THYME LEAVES, DRIED EUCALYPTUS LEAVES, AND WATER.

2. BRING THE MIXTURE TO A BOIL, THEN REDUCE THE HEAT TO LOW AND LET IT SIMMER FOR ABOUT 10 MINUTES.

3. REMOVE THE SAUCEPAN FROM HEAT AND LET THE MIXTURE COOL FOR A FEW MINUTES.

4. STRAIN THE LIQUID INTO A CLEAN JAR OR BOWL, DISCARDING THE HERBS.

5. IF DESIRED, ADD HONEY AND/OR LEMON JUICE TO THE STRAINED LIQUID, STIRRING UNTIL WELL COMBINED.

6. TRANSFER THE RESPIRATORY TONIC INTO A CLEAN, AIRTIGHT JAR AND STORE IT IN THE REFRIGERATOR.

<u>**TO USE THE RESPIRATORY TONIC:**</u>

- TAKE 1-2 TABLESPOONS OF THE TONIC 2-3 TIMES A DAY, OR AS NEEDED FOR RESPIRATORY SUPPORT.

- YOU CAN TAKE THE TONIC DIRECTLY FROM THE SPOON OR MIX IT INTO A HOT DRINK LIKE HERBAL TEA FOR ADDED COMFORT.

- IF USING HONEY AND/OR LEMON JUICE, ADJUST THE AMOUNTS ACCORDING TO YOUR PREFERENCE FOR TASTE.

NOTE: THYME AND EUCALYPTUS ARE GENERALLY SAFE FOR MOST PEOPLE, BUT IT'S ALWAYS A GOOD IDEA TO CONSULT A HEALTHCARE PROFESSIONAL BEFORE USING THEM, ESPECIALLY IF YOU HAVE ANY UNDERLYING HEALTH CONDITIONS, ARE ON MEDICATION, OR IF YOU ARE PREGNANT OR BREASTFEEDING. ADDITIONALLY, IF YOUR RESPIRATORY SYMPTOMS PERSIST OR WORSEN, SEEK MEDICAL ADVICE.

4.4 <u>SLEEP AND RELAXATION</u>

LAVENDER AND CHAMOMILE ARE BOTH POPULAR HERBS KNOWN FOR THEIR CALMING AND RELAXING PROPERTIES. THEY CAN HELP PROMOTE BETTER SLEEP AND ALLEVIATE INSOMNIA. CREATING A SLEEP AID WITH LAVENDER AND CHAMOMILE IS A NATURAL AND EFFECTIVE WAY TO SUPPORT A RESTFUL NIGHT'S SLEEP. HERE'S A RECIPE FOR A LAVENDER AND CHAMOMILE SLEEP AID:

<u>INGREDIENTS:</u>

- 2 TABLESPOONS DRIED LAVENDER FLOWERS

- 2 TABLESPOONS DRIED CHAMOMILE FLOWERS

- 2 CUPS WATER

- 1 TABLESPOON HONEY (OPTIONAL)

<u>INSTRUCTIONS:</u>

1. IN A SMALL SAUCEPAN, COMBINE THE DRIED LAVENDER FLOWERS, DRIED CHAMOMILE FLOWERS, AND WATER.

2. BRING THE MIXTURE TO A BOIL, THEN REDUCE THE HEAT TO LOW AND LET IT SIMMER FOR ABOUT 10 MINUTES.

3. REMOVE THE SAUCEPAN FROM HEAT AND LET THE MIXTURE COOL FOR A FEW MINUTES.

4. STRAIN THE LIQUID INTO A CLEAN JAR OR BOWL, DISCARDING THE HERBS.

5. IF DESIRED, ADD HONEY TO THE STRAINED LIQUID, STIRRING UNTIL WELL COMBINED.

6. TRANSFER THE SLEEP AID INTO A CLEAN, AIRTIGHT JAR AND STORE IT IN A COOL, DARK PLACE.

TO USE THE SLEEP AID:

- DRINK A CUP OF THE SLEEP AID ABOUT 30 MINUTES BEFORE BEDTIME.

- YOU CAN DRINK IT AS IS OR MIX IT WITH WARM MILK OR YOUR FAVORITE HERBAL TEA FOR ADDED RELAXATION.

- ADJUST THE AMOUNT OF HONEY ACCORDING TO YOUR PREFERENCE FOR TASTE.

- TAKE CARE NOT TO CONSUME TOO CLOSE TO BEDTIME, AS IT MAY LEAD TO FREQUENT URINATION DURING THE NIGHT.

VALERIAN AND PASSIONFLOWER ARE TWO HERBS KNOWN FOR THEIR CALMING PROPERTIES AND ABILITY TO REDUCE ANXIETY AND PROMOTE RELAXATION. COMBINING THESE TWO HERBS IN A CALMING ELIXIR CAN HELP YOU UNWIND AND DE-STRESS AFTER A LONG DAY. HERE'S A RECIPE FOR A VALERIAN AND PASSIONFLOWER CALMING ELIXIR:

INGREDIENTS:

- 1 TABLESPOON DRIED VALERIAN ROOT

- 1 TABLESPOON DRIED PASSIONFLOWER

- 2 CUPS WATER

- 1 TABLESPOON HONEY (OPTIONAL)

<u>**INSTRUCTIONS:**</u>

1. IN A SMALL SAUCEPAN, COMBINE THE DRIED VALERIAN ROOT, DRIED PASSIONFLOWER, AND WATER.

2. BRING THE MIXTURE TO A BOIL, THEN REDUCE THE HEAT TO LOW, AND LET IT SIMMER FOR ABOUT 10 MINUTES.

3. REMOVE THE SAUCEPAN FROM HEAT AND LET THE MIXTURE COOL FOR A FEW MINUTES.

4. STRAIN THE LIQUID INTO A CLEAN JAR OR BOWL, DISCARDING THE HERBS.

5. IF DESIRED, ADD HONEY TO THE STRAINED LIQUID, STIRRING UNTIL WELL COMBINED.

6. TRANSFER THE ELIXIR INTO A CLEAN, AIRTIGHT JAR AND STORE IT IN A COOL, DARK PLACE.

<u>**TO USE THE CALMING ELIXIR:**</u>

- DRINK A CUP OF THE ELIXIR ABOUT 30 MINUTES BEFORE BEDTIME OR WHENEVER YOU NEED TO RELAX.

- YOU CAN DRINK IT AS IS OR MIX IT WITH WARM WATER, TEA, OR JUICE FOR ADDED FLAVOR.

- ADJUST THE AMOUNT OF HONEY ACCORDING TO YOUR PREFERENCE FOR TASTE.

- TAKE CARE NOT TO CONSUME TOO CLOSE TO BEDTIME IF YOU NEED TO WAKE UP EARLY, AS VALERIAN MAY CAUSE DROWSINESS.

NOTE: VALERIAN AND PASSIONFLOWER ARE GENERALLY SAFE FOR MOST PEOPLE, BUT IT'S ALWAYS A GOOD IDEA TO CONSULT A HEALTHCARE PROFESSIONAL BEFORE USING THEM, ESPECIALLY IF YOU HAVE ANY UNDERLYING HEALTH CONDITIONS, ARE ON MEDICATION, OR IF YOU ARE PREGNANT OR BREASTFEEDING. ADDITIONALLY, IF YOUR ANXIETY OR SLEEP PROBLEMS PERSIST OR WORSEN, SEEK MEDICAL ADVICE.

4.5 <u>ENERGY AND VITALITY</u>

GINSENG AND MACA ARE TWO HERBS KNOWN FOR THEIR ENERGY-BOOSTING PROPERTIES AND ABILITY TO ENHANCE PHYSICAL AND MENTAL STAMINA. COMBINING THESE TWO HERBS IN AN ENERGIZING TINCTURE CAN HELP IMPROVE FOCUS, INCREASE VITALITY, AND COMBAT FATIGUE. HERE'S A RECIPE FOR A GINSENG AND MACA ENERGIZING TINCTURE:

INGREDIENTS:

- 1 TABLESPOON DRIED GINSENG ROOT

- 1 TABLESPOON DRIED MACA ROOT

- 1 CUP VODKA OR HIGH-PROOF ALCOHOL

INSTRUCTIONS:

1. IN A GLASS JAR, COMBINE THE DRIED GINSENG ROOT, DRIED MACA ROOT, AND VODKA (OR HIGH-PROOF ALCOHOL) UNTIL THE HERBS ARE COMPLETELY COVERED.

2. SEAL THE JAR TIGHTLY AND SHAKE IT VIGOROUSLY TO ENSURE THE HERBS ARE WELL MIXED WITH THE ALCOHOL.

3. PLACE THE JAR IN A COOL, DARK PLACE AND LET THE MIXTURE STEEP FOR 4-6 WEEKS. SHAKE THE JAR OCCASIONALLY DURING THIS TIME.

4. AFTER THE STEEPING PERIOD, STRAIN THE LIQUID INTO A CLEAN, DARK-COLORED GLASS DROPPER BOTTLE. DISCARD THE HERBS.

5. STORE THE TINCTURE IN A COOL, DARK PLACE.

<u>**TO USE THE ENERGIZING TINCTURE:**</u>

- TAKE 1-2 DROPPERFULS (ABOUT 30-60 DROPS) OF THE TINCTURE ONCE OR TWICE A DAY.

- YOU CAN TAKE IT DIRECTLY UNDER THE TONGUE OR MIX IT WITH A SMALL AMOUNT OF WATER, TEA, OR JUICE.

- START WITH A LOWER DOSAGE AND GRADUALLY INCREASE IF NEEDED, AS EVERYONE RESPONDS DIFFERENTLY TO HERBAL REMEDIES.

- IT'S RECOMMENDED TO TAKE THE TINCTURE IN THE MORNING OR EARLY AFTERNOON TO AVOID DISRUPTING SLEEP.

NOTE: GINSENG AND MACA MAY INTERACT WITH CERTAIN MEDICATIONS OR HEALTH CONDITIONS, SO IT'S ESSENTIAL TO CONSULT A HEALTHCARE PROFESSIONAL BEFORE USING THEM, ESPECIALLY IF YOU HAVE ANY UNDERLYING HEALTH CONDITIONS OR IF YOU ARE PREGNANT OR BREASTFEEDING. ADDITIONALLY, IF YOU EXPERIENCE ANY ADVERSE EFFECTS OR HAVE ANY CONCERNS, DISCONTINUE USE AND CONSULT A HEALTHCARE PROFESSIONAL.

NETTLE AND ASHWAGANDHA ARE TWO POWERFUL HERBS THAT CAN HELP REVITALIZE THE BODY AND PROMOTE OVERALL WELL-BEING. NETTLE IS RICH IN VITAMINS AND MINERALS, WHILE ASHWAGANDHA IS KNOWN FOR ITS ADAPTOGENIC PROPERTIES THAT HELP THE BODY MANAGE STRESS. TOGETHER, THEY CREATE A REVITALIZING BLEND THAT CAN SUPPORT ENERGY LEVELS AND ENHANCE VITALITY. HERE'S A RECIPE FOR A NETTLE AND ASHWAGANDHA REVITALIZING BLEND:

INGREDIENTS:

- 2 TABLESPOONS DRIED NETTLE LEAVES

- 1 TABLESPOON DRIED ASHWAGANDHA ROOT

- 1 CUP HOT WATER

- HONEY OR LEMON (OPTIONAL, FOR TASTE)

INSTRUCTIONS:

1. IN A TEAPOT OR HEATPROOF CONTAINER, COMBINE THE DRIED NETTLE LEAVES AND ASHWAGANDHA ROOT.

2. POUR THE HOT WATER OVER THE HERBS AND COVER THE CONTAINER. LET IT STEEP FOR 15-20 MINUTES.

3. ONCE STEEPED, STRAIN THE MIXTURE TO REMOVE THE HERBS. YOU CAN USE A FINE-MESH STRAINER OR A TEA INFUSER.

4. OPTIONAL: ADD HONEY OR LEMON TO TASTE, IF DESIRED.

5. POUR THE REVITALIZING BLEND INTO A CUP AND ENJOY.

<u>TO USE THE REVITALIZING BLEND:</u>

- DRINK 1-2 CUPS DAILY.

- YOU CAN CONSUME THE BLEND IN THE MORNING TO KICKSTART YOUR DAY OR AS A MID-DAY PICK-ME-UP.

- ADJUST THE AMOUNT OF HERBS USED ACCORDING TO YOUR PREFERENCE. YOU CAN INCREASE OR DECREASE THE QUANTITIES TO SUIT YOUR TASTE.

- IF YOU PREFER A STRONGER FLAVOR OR MORE POTENT BLEND, YOU CAN INCREASE THE STEEPING TIME.

NOTE: IT'S ALWAYS ADVISABLE TO CONSULT A HEALTHCARE PROFESSIONAL BEFORE USING ANY HERBAL REMEDIES, ESPECIALLY IF YOU HAVE ANY UNDERLYING HEALTH CONDITIONS OR IF YOU ARE PREGNANT OR BREASTFEEDING. IF YOU EXPERIENCE ANY ADVERSE EFFECTS OR HAVE ANY CONCERNS, DISCONTINUE USE AND CONSULT A HEALTHCARE PROFESSIONAL.

4.6 **STRESS AND ANXIETY RELIEF**

LEMON BALM AND SKULLCAP ARE TWO HERBS WITH CALMING PROPERTIES THAT CAN HELP PROMOTE RELAXATION AND REDUCE STRESS. LEMON BALM IS KNOWN FOR ITS SOOTHING EFFECTS ON THE NERVOUS SYSTEM, WHILE SKULLCAP IS A NERVINE HERB THAT HELPS CALM THE MIND. TOGETHER, THEY CREATE A STRESS-RELIEVING ELIXIR THAT CAN HELP YOU UNWIND AND FIND A SENSE OF PEACE. HERE'S A RECIPE FOR A LEMON BALM AND SKULLCAP STRESS-RELIEVING ELIXIR:

INGREDIENTS:

- 2 TABLESPOONS DRIED LEMON BALM LEAVES

- 1 TABLESPOON DRIED SKULLCAP LEAVES

- 1 CUP HOT WATER

- HONEY OR STEVIA (OPTIONAL, FOR TASTE)

INSTRUCTIONS:

1. IN A TEAPOT OR HEATPROOF CONTAINER, COMBINE THE DRIED LEMON BALM AND SKULLCAP LEAVES.

2. POUR THE HOT WATER OVER THE HERBS AND COVER THE CONTAINER. LET IT STEEP FOR 15-20 MINUTES.

3. ONCE STEEPED, STRAIN THE MIXTURE TO REMOVE THE LEAVES. YOU CAN USE A FINE-MESH STRAINER OR A TEA INFUSER.

4. OPTIONAL: ADD HONEY OR STEVIA TO TASTE, IF DESIRED.

5. POUR THE STRESS-RELIEVING ELIXIR INTO A CUP AND ENJOY

<u>TO USE THE STRESS-RELIEVING ELIXIR:</u>

- DRINK 1-2 CUPS DAILY.

- YOU CAN CONSUME THE ELIXIR IN THE EVENING TO HELP YOU RELAX BEFORE BED OR DURING TIMES OF HIGH STRESS.

- ADJUST THE AMOUNT OF HERBS USED ACCORDING TO YOUR PREFERENCE. YOU CAN INCREASE OR DECREASE THE QUANTITIES TO SUIT YOUR TASTE.

- IF YOU PREFER A STRONGER FLAVOR OR MORE POTENT ELIXIR, YOU CAN INCREASE THE STEEPING TIME.

NOTE: IT'S ALWAYS ADVISABLE TO CONSULT A HEALTHCARE PROFESSIONAL BEFORE USING ANY HERBAL REMEDIES, ESPECIALLY IF YOU HAVE ANY UNDERLYING HEALTH CONDITIONS OR IF YOU ARE PREGNANT OR BREASTFEEDING. IF YOU EXPERIENCE ANY ADVERSE EFFECTS OR HAVE ANY CONCERNS, DISCONTINUE USE AND CONSULT A HEALTHCARE PROFESSIONAL.

HOLY BASIL AND ASHWAGANDHA ARE TWO POWERFUL ADAPTOGENIC HERBS KNOWN FOR THEIR ABILITY TO HELP THE BODY ADAPT TO STRESS AND PROMOTE OVERALL WELL-BEING. MAKING A TINCTURE WITH THESE HERBS ALLOWS YOU TO CONVENIENTLY HARNESS THEIR BENEFITS. HERE'S A RECIPE FOR A HOLY BASIL AND ASHWAGANDHA ADAPTOGEN TINCTURE:

INGREDIENTS:

- 1 CUP DRIED HOLY BASIL LEAVES

- 1 CUP DRIED ASHWAGANDHA ROOT

- 2 CUPS HIGH-PROOF ALCOHOL (SUCH AS VODKA OR BRANDY)

INSTRUCTIONS:

1. IN A GLASS JAR WITH A TIGHT-FITTING LID, COMBINE THE DRIED HOLY BASIL LEAVES AND ASHWAGANDHA ROOT.

2. POUR THE HIGH-PROOF ALCOHOL OVER THE HERBS, MAKING SURE THEY ARE FULLY SUBMERGED.

3. SEAL THE JAR TIGHTLY, AND STORE IT IN A COOL, DARK PLACE FOR 4-6 WEEKS. SHAKE THE JAR GENTLY EVERY FEW DAYS TO HELP EXTRACT THE PROPERTIES FROM THE HERBS.

4. AFTER THE STEEPING PERIOD, STRAIN THE MIXTURE THROUGH A FINE-MESH STRAINER OR CHEESECLOTH TO REMOVE THE HERBS.

5. TRANSFER THE TINCTURE INTO AMBER GLASS DROPPER BOTTLES FOR STORAGE.

TO USE THE ADAPTOGEN TINCTURE:

- TAKE 30-60 DROPS (ABOUT 1-2 DROPPERS FULL) UP TO THREE TIMES DAILY.

- YOU CAN CONSUME THE TINCTURE DIRECTLY OR MIX IT WITH WATER, JUICE, OR TEA FOR EASIER CONSUMPTION.

- START WITH A LOWER DOSAGE AND GRADUALLY INCREASE IT IF NEEDED, BASED ON YOUR BODY'S RESPONSE.

- THE TINCTURE CAN BE TAKEN AS NEEDED DURING TIMES OF STRESS OR REGULARLY ON A DAILY BASIS FOR LONG-TERM SUPPORT.

NOTE: IT'S IMPORTANT TO CONSULT A HEALTHCARE PROFESSIONAL BEFORE USING ANY HERBAL REMEDIES, ESPECIALLY IF YOU HAVE ANY UNDERLYING HEALTH CONDITIONS OR IF YOU ARE PREGNANT OR BREASTFEEDING. THEY CAN PROVIDE GUIDANCE ON APPROPRIATE DOSAGES AND POTENTIAL INTERACTIONS WITH ANY MEDICATIONS

YOU MAY BE TAKING. IF YOU EXPERIENCE ANY ADVERSE EFFECTS OR HAVE ANY CONCERNS, DISCONTINUE USE AND SEEK ADVICE FROM A HEALTHCARE PROFESSIONAL.

BRINGING HOLISTIC WELLNESS INTO YOUR DAILY ROUTINE INVOLVES TAKING A COMPREHENSIVE APPROACH TO YOUR PHYSICAL, MENTAL, AND EMOTIONAL WELL-BEING.

HERE ARE SOME TIPS TO HELP YOU INCORPORATE HOLISTIC PRACTICES INTO YOUR DAILY LIFE:

1. **<u>START YOUR DAY WITH INTENTION</u>:** BEGIN EACH MORNING BY SETTING A POSITIVE INTENTION FOR THE DAY. THIS COULD BE A MANTRA, AFFIRMATION, OR GOAL YOU WANT TO FOCUS ON.

2. **<u>MINDFUL EATING</u>:** PAY ATTENTION TO WHAT AND HOW YOU EAT. CHOOSE WHOLE, NOURISHING FOODS THAT SUPPORT YOUR BODY'S NEEDS. PRACTICE MINDFUL EATING BY SAVORING EACH BITE, EATING SLOWLY, AND LISTENING TO YOUR BODY'S HUNGER AND FULLNESS CUES.

3. **<u>STAY ACTIVE</u>:** INCORPORATE REGULAR PHYSICAL ACTIVITY INTO YOUR ROUTINE. CHOOSE ACTIVITIES YOU ENJOY, SUCH AS YOGA, WALKING, DANCING, OR SWIMMING. EXERCISE NOT ONLY BENEFITS YOUR PHYSICAL HEALTH BUT ALSO RELEASES

ENDORPHINS, IMPROVING YOUR MOOD AND REDUCING STRESS.

4. **<u>PRACTICE SELF-CARE</u>:** MAKE TIME FOR SELF-CARE ACTIVITIES THAT NURTURE YOUR MIND, BODY, AND SOUL. THIS COULD INCLUDE TAKING BATHS, READING, JOURNALING, PRACTICING MEDITATION OR DEEP BREATHING EXERCISES, OR ENGAGING IN HOBBIES YOU ENJOY.

5. **<u>CONNECT WITH NATURE</u>:** SPEND TIME OUTDOORS AND CONNECT WITH THE NATURAL WORLD. THIS COULD INVOLVE GOING FOR WALKS IN NATURE, GARDENING, OR SIMPLY SITTING IN A PARK OR GARDEN. NATURE HAS A CALMING EFFECT ON THE MIND AND CAN HELP RELIEVE STRESS.

6. **<u>PRIORITIZE SLEEP</u>:** AIM FOR CONSISTENT AND SUFFICIENT SLEEP EACH NIGHT. CREATE A SLEEP-FRIENDLY ENVIRONMENT, ESTABLISH A BEDTIME ROUTINE, AND LIMIT SCREEN TIME BEFORE BED TO ENSURE RESTORATIVE REST.

7. **<u>NURTURE YOUR RELATIONSHIPS</u>:** FOSTER POSITIVE RELATIONSHIPS WITH LOVED ONES BY SPENDING QUALITY

TIME TOGETHER, EXPRESSING GRATITUDE, AND PRACTICING EFFECTIVE COMMUNICATION. SURROUND YOURSELF WITH PEOPLE WHO SUPPORT AND UPLIFT YOU.

8. **<u>PRACTICE MINDFULNESS:</u>** PAY ATTENTION TO THE PRESENT MOMENT AND CULTIVATE MINDFULNESS THROUGHOUT THE DAY. THIS CAN HELP REDUCE STRESS, INCREASE SELF-AWARENESS, AND ENHANCE YOUR OVERALL WELL-BEING.

9. **<u>SEEK HOLISTIC THERAPIES:</u>** CONSIDER EXPLORING VARIOUS HOLISTIC THERAPIES, SUCH AS ACUPUNCTURE, MASSAGE, AROMATHERAPY, OR HERBAL REMEDIES, THAT CAN SUPPORT YOUR OVERALL HEALTH AND BALANCE.

10. **<u>LISTEN TO YOUR BODY:</u>** TUNE IN TO YOUR BODY'S SIGNALS AND NEEDS. REST WHEN YOU'RE TIRED, NOURISH YOURSELF WITH HEALTHY FOOD, AND ENGAGE IN ACTIVITIES THAT BRING YOU JOY AND FULFILLMENT.

REMEMBER, HOLISTIC WELLNESS IS ABOUT FINDING BALANCE AND HARMONY IN ALL ASPECTS OF YOUR LIFE. IT'S ABOUT TAKING CARE OF YOUR PHYSICAL, MENTAL, AND

EMOTIONAL WELL-BEING TO LEAD A FULFILLING AND VIBRANT LIFE. EXPERIMENT WITH DIFFERENT PRACTICES AND TECHNIQUES TO FIND WHAT WORKS BEST FOR YOU, AND ALWAYS LISTEN TO YOUR BODY'S WISDOM.

WHEN SOURCING HIGH-QUALITY HERBS FOR HOLISTIC WELLNESS, IT'S IMPORTANT TO CONSIDER THE FOLLOWING TIPS: *BY FOLLOWING THESE TIPS, YOU CAN INCREASE YOUR CHANCES OF SOURCING HIGH-QUALITY HERBS THAT WILL SUPPORT YOUR HOLISTIC WELLNESS JOURNEY.*

1. **<u>RESEARCH THE SOURCE</u>:** LOOK FOR REPUTABLE SUPPLIERS OR COMPANIES THAT PRIORITIZE QUALITY, SUSTAINABILITY, AND ETHICAL SOURCING PRACTICES. READ REVIEWS, CHECK THEIR CERTIFICATIONS OR MEMBERSHIPS, AND LEARN ABOUT THEIR FARMING OR HARVESTING METHODS.

2. **<u>ORGANIC CERTIFICATION</u>:** CHOOSE HERBS THAT ARE CERTIFIED ORGANIC. THIS ENSURES THAT THE HERBS WERE GROWN WITHOUT THE USE OF SYNTHETIC PESTICIDES, HERBICIDES, OR OTHER CHEMICALS THAT CAN BE HARMFUL TO YOUR HEALTH.

3. **WILDCRAFTED OR ETHICALLY SOURCED**: SOME HERBS ARE WILDCRAFTED, MEANING THEY ARE HARVESTED FROM THEIR NATURAL HABITATS. LOOK FOR SUPPLIERS THAT ETHICALLY AND SUSTAINABLY WILDCRAFT THEIR HERBS, ENSURING THEY ARE NOT OVER-HARVESTED AND THAT THEIR COLLECTION PRACTICES HAVE MINIMAL IMPACT ON THE ENVIRONMENT.

4. **TESTING AND QUALITY CONTROL**: SELECT SUPPLIERS THAT CONDUCT THIRD-PARTY TESTING TO VERIFY THE QUALITY AND PURITY OF THEIR HERBS. LOOK FOR COMPANIES THAT PROVIDE BATCH-SPECIFIC TEST RESULTS FOR THINGS LIKE HEAVY METALS, PESTICIDES, AND MICROBIAL CONTAMINATION.

5. **FRESHNESS AND STORAGE**: OPT FOR HERBS THAT ARE FRESH AND HAVE A STRONG AROMA. A REPUTABLE SUPPLIER WILL ENSURE PROPER STORAGE AND HANDLING TO MAINTAIN THE HERB'S POTENCY AND QUALITY.

6. **<u>INFORMATION TRANSPARENCY</u>:** CHOOSE SUPPLIERS THAT PROVIDE DETAILED INFORMATION ABOUT THE HERB'S ORIGIN, CULTIVATION METHODS, AND ANY TESTING OR CERTIFICATIONS THEY HAVE. THIS DEMONSTRATES TRANSPARENCY AND A COMMITMENT TO QUALITY.

7. **<u>SUSTAINABLE PACKAGING</u>:** LOOK FOR SUPPLIERS THAT USE ECO-FRIENDLY AND SUSTAINABLE PACKAGING MATERIALS TO MINIMIZE THEIR ENVIRONMENTAL IMPACT.

8. **<u>CONSIDER LOCAL OPTIONS</u>:** WHENEVER POSSIBLE, SUPPORT LOCAL HERB GROWERS AND FARMERS' MARKETS. THIS ALLOWS YOU TO HAVE DIRECT CONTACT WITH THE PRODUCERS, ENSURING FRESHNESS AND SUPPORTING YOUR LOCAL COMMUNITY.

9. **<u>EDUCATE YOURSELF</u>:** LEARN ABOUT THE HERB YOU ARE INTERESTED IN, ITS CHARACTERISTICS, AND THE BEST WAYS TO IDENTIFY HIGH-QUALITY SPECIMENS. THIS KNOWLEDGE WILL HELP YOU MAKE INFORMED DECISIONS WHEN PURCHASING HERBS.

10. **<u>TRUST YOUR INSTINCTS</u>:** ULTIMATELY, TRUST YOUR INSTINCTS AND INTUITION WHEN CHOOSING HERBS. IF SOMETHING DOESN'T FEEL RIGHT OR IF THE QUALITY SEEMS QUESTIONABLE, EXPLORE OTHER OPTIONS.

INCORPORATING HERBAL TINCTURES INTO A HEALTHIER LIFESTYLE CAN PROVIDE A RANGE OF BENEFITS. HERE ARE SOME TIPS FOR INTEGRATING THEM:

1. **<u>RESEARCH AND CHOOSE THE RIGHT HERBS</u>:** DETERMINE WHICH HERBS ALIGN WITH YOUR SPECIFIC HEALTH GOALS. WHETHER IT'S SUPPORTING IMMUNE HEALTH, IMPROVING DIGESTION, PROMOTING RELAXATION, OR ADDRESSING OTHER CONCERNS, SELECT TINCTURES THAT CONTAIN THE HERBS THAT ARE MOST BENEFICIAL FOR YOU.

2. **<u>START WITH ONE OR TWO TINCTURES</u>:** IT'S BEST TO BEGIN WITH ONE OR TWO TINCTURES TO OBSERVE HOW YOUR BODY RESPONDS. THIS ALLOWS YOU TO ASSESS THEIR EFFICACY AND DETERMINE IF ANY ADJUSTMENTS ARE NEEDED.

3. **<u>CONSULT WITH A HEALTHCARE PROFESSIONAL</u>:** IF YOU HAVE SPECIFIC HEALTH CONDITIONS OR ARE TAKING MEDICATIONS, CONSULT WITH A HEALTHCARE PROFESSIONAL, SUCH AS AN HERBALIST OR NATUROPATHIC DOCTOR. THEY CAN PROVIDE GUIDANCE ON THE APPROPRIATE HERBS AND DOSAGES FOR YOUR SITUATION.

4. **<u>FOLLOW RECOMMENDED DOSAGES</u>:** EACH TINCTURE WILL HAVE ITS RECOMMENDED DOSAGE INSTRUCTIONS. IT'S IMPORTANT TO ADHERE TO THESE GUIDELINES TO ENSURE THE PROPER BALANCE AND EFFECTIVENESS.

5. **<u>CREATE A ROUTINE</u>:** INCORPORATE THE TINCTURES INTO YOUR DAILY ROUTINE BY TAKING THEM AT CONSISTENT TIMES. THIS CAN HELP ESTABLISH A HABIT AND ENSURE REGULAR CONSUMPTION.

6. **<u>USE THEM AS DIRECTED</u>:** SOME TINCTURES MAY NEED TO BE DILUTED IN WATER OR TAKEN WITH FOOD, WHILE OTHERS CAN BE TAKEN DIRECTLY UNDER THE TONGUE. READ THE INSTRUCTIONS CAREFULLY AND FOLLOW THEM TO ENSURE MAXIMUM EFFECTIVENESS.

7. **<u>BE PATIENT</u>:** HERBAL TINCTURES MAY TAKE TIME TO SHOW THEIR EFFECTS. STAY CONSISTENT WITH YOUR ROUTINE AND GIVE THEM TIME TO WORK. IT'S ALSO WORTH NOTING THAT INDIVIDUAL RESPONSES MAY VARY, SO WHAT WORKS FOR ONE PERSON MAY NOT BE THE SAME FOR ANOTHER.

8. **<u>OBSERVE AND EVALUATE</u>:** PAY ATTENTION TO ANY CHANGES OR IMPROVEMENTS IN YOUR WELL-BEING. KEEP TRACK OF YOUR EXPERIENCES AND ADJUST YOUR DOSAGE OR CHOICE OF HERBS IF NECESSARY.

9. **<u>COMBINE WITH OTHER HEALTHY HABITS</u>:** INCORPORATE HERBAL TINCTURES INTO A HOLISTIC APPROACH TO WELLNESS. THIS CAN INCLUDE MAINTAINING A BALANCED DIET, REGULAR EXERCISE, QUALITY SLEEP, STRESS MANAGEMENT, AND OTHER LIFESTYLE PRACTICES THAT SUPPORT YOUR OVERALL WELL-BEING.

10. **<u>EDUCATE YOURSELF</u>:** CONTINUOUSLY LEARN ABOUT HERBS AND THEIR BENEFITS. UNDERSTAND THE PROPER USE AND POTENTIAL INTERACTIONS WITH MEDICATIONS OR HEALTH CONDITIONS. THIS KNOWLEDGE EMPOWERS YOU TO MAKE INFORMED DECISIONS AND GET THE MOST OUT OF YOUR HERBAL TINCTURES.

- *REMEMBER, HERBAL TINCTURES ARE NOT A SUBSTITUTE FOR PROFESSIONAL MEDICAL ADVICE. IF YOU HAVE ANY CONCERNS ABOUT YOUR HEALTH, IT'S ALWAYS BEST TO CONSULT WITH A QUALIFIED HEALTHCARE PROVIDER.*

APPENDIX:

THERE ARE NUMEROUS HERBAL TINCTURES AVAILABLE, EACH WITH THEIR OWN UNIQUE BENEFITS AND USES. HERE IS AN OVERVIEW OF SOME COMMONLY USED HERBAL TINCTURES:

1. **ECHINACEA:** KNOWN FOR ITS IMMUNE-BOOSTING PROPERTIES, ECHINACEA TINCTURE IS OFTEN USED TO PREVENT AND ALLEVIATE SYMPTOMS OF THE COMMON COLD AND OTHER UPPER RESPIRATORY TRACT INFECTIONS.

2. **MILK THISTLE**: MILK THISTLE TINCTURE IS DERIVED FROM THE SEEDS OF THE MILK THISTLE PLANT. IT IS COMMONLY USED TO SUPPORT LIVER HEALTH AND PROMOTE DETOXIFICATION.

3. **VALERIAN**: VALERIAN ROOT TINCTURE IS OFTEN USED AS A NATURAL REMEDY FOR INSOMNIA AND SLEEP DISORDERS. IT HAS CALMING PROPERTIES THAT CAN HELP PROMOTE RELAXATION AND IMPROVE SLEEP QUALITY.

4. **<u>ST. JOHN'S WORT</u>**: ST. JOHN'S WORT TINCTURE IS COMMONLY USED TO RELIEVE SYMPTOMS OF MILD TO MODERATE DEPRESSION AND ANXIETY. IT MAY ALSO HELP ALLEVIATE SYMPTOMS OF SEASONAL AFFECTIVE DISORDER (SAD).

5. **<u>GINGER</u>**: GINGER TINCTURE IS KNOWN FOR ITS ANTI-INFLAMMATORY AND DIGESTIVE PROPERTIES. IT CAN HELP ALLEVIATE NAUSEA, INDIGESTION, AND SUPPORT OVERALL DIGESTIVE HEALTH.

6. **<u>CHAMOMILE</u>**: CHAMOMILE TINCTURE IS WIDELY USED FOR ITS CALMING EFFECTS AND IS OFTEN USED TO PROMOTE RELAXATION AND REDUCE ANXIETY. IT CAN ALSO HELP WITH DIGESTIVE ISSUES AND PROMOTE HEALTHY SLEEP.

7. **<u>TURMERIC</u>**: TURMERIC TINCTURE IS DERIVED FROM THE ROOT OF THE TURMERIC PLANT AND CONTAINS THE ACTIVE COMPOUND CURCUMIN, KNOWN FOR ITS POTENT ANTI-INFLAMMATORY PROPERTIES. IT IS USED TO SUPPORT JOINT HEALTH, REDUCE INFLAMMATION, AND PROMOTE OVERALL WELL-BEING.

8. **HAWTHORN:** HAWTHORN TINCTURE IS DERIVED FROM THE BERRIES, LEAVES, AND FLOWERS OF THE HAWTHORN PLANT. IT IS COMMONLY USED TO SUPPORT CARDIOVASCULAR HEALTH, REGULATE BLOOD PRESSURE, AND IMPROVE CIRCULATION.

9. **PASSIONFLOWER:** PASSIONFLOWER TINCTURE IS OFTEN USED FOR ITS CALMING AND SEDATIVE EFFECTS. IT CAN HELP REDUCE ANXIETY AND PROMOTE RESTFUL SLEEP.

10. **LEMON BALM:** LEMON BALM TINCTURE IS DERIVED FROM THE LEAVES OF THE LEMON BALM PLANT. IT IS COMMONLY USED TO RELIEVE STRESS, ANXIETY, AND PROMOTE RELAXATION. IT MAY ALSO HELP IMPROVE COGNITIVE FUNCTION AND SUPPORT DIGESTIVE HEALTH.

11. **NETTLE:** NETTLE TINCTURE IS DERIVED FROM THE LEAVES OF THE NETTLE PLANT. IT IS RICH IN VITAMINS AND MINERALS AND IS OFTEN USED TO SUPPORT ALLERGIES, JOINT HEALTH, AND OVERALL WELLNESS.

1. <u>**ECHINACEA**</u>:

- **INDICATIONS:** BOOSTING IMMUNE SYSTEM, PREVENTING AND ALLEVIATING SYMPTOMS OF THE COMMON COLD AND OTHER UPPER RESPIRATORY TRACT INFECTIONS.

- **DOSAGE:** ADULTS CAN TAKE 2-3 ML OF ECHINACEA TINCTURE, 2-3 TIMES A DAY. CHILDREN SHOULD TAKE A LOWER DOSAGE BASED ON THEIR AGE AND WEIGHT.

- **PRECAUTIONS:** AVOID USING ECHINACEA TINCTURE FOR MORE THAN 8 WEEKS AT A TIME. IT MAY INTERFERE WITH SOME MEDICATIONS, SO CONSULT WITH A HEALTHCARE PROFESSIONAL IF YOU ARE TAKING ANY MEDICATIONS OR HAVE ANY UNDERLYING HEALTH CONDITIONS.

2. <u>**MILK THISTLE**</u>:

- **INDICATIONS:** SUPPORTING LIVER HEALTH, PROMOTING DETOXIFICATION.

- **DOSAGE:** TAKE 2-3 ML OF MILK THISTLE TINCTURE, 2-3 TIMES A DAY.

- **PRECAUTIONS:** CONSULT WITH A HEALTHCARE PROFESSIONAL IF YOU HAVE ANY LIVER CONDITIONS OR ARE TAKING MEDICATIONS THAT MAY INTERACT WITH MILK THISTLE.

3. <u>**VALERIAN:**</u>

- **INDICATIONS**: PROMOTING RELAXATION, IMPROVING SLEEP QUALITY.

- **DOSAGE:** TAKE 2-3 ML OF VALERIAN TINCTURE, 1-2 HOURS BEFORE BED.

- **PRECAUTIONS:** AVOID DRIVING OR OPERATING HEAVY MACHINERY AFTER TAKING VALERIAN. IT MAY CAUSE DROWSINESS OR IMPAIR YOUR ABILITY TO PERFORM TASKS REQUIRING ALERTNESS.

4. <u>**ST. JOHN'S WORT:**</u>

- **INDICATIONS:** RELIEVING SYMPTOMS OF MILD TO MODERATE DEPRESSION AND ANXIETY, ALLEVIATING SYMPTOMS OF SEASONAL AFFECTIVE DISORDER (SAD).

- **DOSAGE:** TAKE 2-4 ML OF ST. JOHN'S WORT TINCTURE, UP TO 3 TIMES A DAY.

- **PRECAUTIONS:** ST. JOHN'S WORT MAY INTERACT WITH CERTAIN MEDICATIONS, INCLUDING BIRTH CONTROL PILLS, ANTIDEPRESSANTS, AND BLOOD THINNERS. CONSULT WITH A HEALTHCARE PROFESSIONAL IF YOU ARE TAKING ANY MEDICATIONS.

5. **GINGER**:

- **INDICATIONS:** REDUCING INFLAMMATION, ALLEVIATING NAUSEA, SUPPORTING DIGESTIVE HEALTH.

- **DOSAGE:** TAKE 2-4 ML OF GINGER TINCTURE, UP TO 3 TIMES A DAY.

- **PRECAUTIONS:** GINGER MAY INCREASE THE RISK OF BLEEDING, SO USE CAUTION IF YOU HAVE A BLEEDING DISORDER OR ARE TAKING BLOOD THINNERS.

6. **CHAMOMILE**:

- **INDICATIONS:** PROMOTING RELAXATION, REDUCING ANXIETY, IMPROVING SLEEP, SUPPORTING DIGESTIVE HEALTH.

- **DOSAGE:** TAKE 3-4 ML OF CHAMOMILE TINCTURE, UP TO 3 TIMES A DAY.

- **PRECAUTIONS:** CHAMOMILE MAY CAUSE DROWSINESS, SO AVOID DRIVING OR OPERATING HEAVY MACHINERY AFTER TAKING IT. CONSULT WITH A HEALTHCARE PROFESSIONAL IF YOU ARE PREGNANT OR BREASTFEEDING.

7. **<u>TURMERIC</u>:**

- **INDICATIONS:** REDUCING INFLAMMATION, SUPPORTING JOINT HEALTH, PROMOTING OVERALL WELL-BEING.

- **DOSAGE:** TAKE 2-3 ML OF TURMERIC TINCTURE, 2-3 TIMES A DAY.

- **PRECAUTIONS:** TURMERIC MAY INTERACT WITH CERTAIN MEDICATIONS, INCLUDING BLOOD THINNERS AND ANTIPLATELET DRUGS. CONSULT WITH A HEALTHCARE PROFESSIONAL IF YOU ARE TAKING ANY MEDICATIONS.

8. **<u>HAWTHORN</u>:**

- **INDICATIONS**: SUPPORTING CARDIOVASCULAR HEALTH, REGULATING BLOOD PRESSURE, IMPROVING CIRCULATION.

- **DOSAGE:** TAKE 2-4 ML OF HAWTHORN TINCTURE, UP TO 3 TIMES A DAY.

- **PRECAUTIONS:** CONSULT WITH A HEALTHCARE PROFESSIONAL IF YOU HAVE ANY HEART CONDITIONS OR ARE TAKING MEDICATIONS THAT MAY INTERACT WITH HAWTHORN.

9. **<u>PASSIONFLOWER</u>:**

- **INDICATIONS:** REDUCING ANXIETY, PROMOTING RESTFUL SLEEP.

- **DOSAGE:** TAKE 2-4 ML OF PASSIONFLOWER TINCTURE, UP TO 3 TIMES A DAY.

- **PRECAUTIONS:** PASSIONFLOWER MAY CAUSE DROWSINESS, SO AVOID DRIVING OR OPERATING HEAVY MACHINERY AFTER TAKING IT. CONSULT WITH A HEALTHCARE PROFESSIONAL IF YOU ARE PREGNANT OR BREASTFEEDING.

10. **<u>LEMON BALM</u>:**

- **INDICATIONS:** RELIEVING STRESS, REDUCING ANXIETY, PROMOTING RELAXATION, IMPROVING COGNITIVE FUNCTION, SUPPORTING DIGESTIVE HEALTH.

- **DOSAGE:** TAKE 2-3 ML OF LEMON BALM TINCTURE, UP TO 3 TIMES A DAY.

- **PRECAUTIONS:** LEMON BALM MAY CAUSE DROWSINESS, SO AVOID DRIVING OR OPERATING HEAVY MACHINERY AFTER TAKING IT. CONSULT WITH A HEALTHCARE PROFESSIONAL IF YOU ARE PREGNANT OR BREASTFEEDING.

11. **<u>NETTLE</u>:**

- **INDICATIONS:** SUPPORTING ALLERGIES, JOINT HEALTH, OVERALL WELLNESS.

- **DOSAGE:** TAKE 2-4 ML OF NETTLE TINCTURE, UP TO 3 TIMES A DAY.

- **PRECAUTIONS:** NETTLE MAY HAVE A DIURETIC EFFECT, SO USE CAUTION IF YOU HAVE KIDNEY OR BLADDER ISSUES. CONSULT WITH A HEALTHCARE PROFESSIONAL IF YOU ARE TAKING ANY MEDICATIONS OR HAVE ANY UNDERLYING HEALTH CONDITIONS.

IT'S IMPORTANT TO NOTE THAT THE DOSAGE AND DURATION OF USE FOR EACH HERBAL TINCTURE MAY VARY. IT IS RECOMMENDED TO CONSULT WITH A HEALTHCARE PROFESSIONAL OR HERBALIST BEFORE INCLUDING HERBAL TINCTURES IN YOUR ROUTINE, ESPECIALLY IF YOU HAVE ANY UNDERLYING HEALTH CONDITIONS OR ARE TAKING MEDICATIONS. THEY CAN PROVIDE PERSONALIZED ADVICE AND GUIDANCE BASED ON YOUR INDIVIDUAL NEEDS.

GLOSSARY:

1. **HERBAL TINCTURE**: A CONCENTRATED HERBAL EXTRACT WHERE RAW PLANT MATERIAL IS SOAKED IN ALCOHOL (USUALLY HIGH-PROOF ALCOHOL) FOR A SPECIFIC PERIOD TO EXTRACT ITS MEDICINAL PROPERTIES.

2. **AILMENT**: A PHYSICAL OR MENTAL CONDITION OR DISEASE THAT CAUSES DISCOMFORT OR DISTRESS TO THE BODY OR MIND.

3. **HOLISTIC**: AN APPROACH THAT EMPHASIZES THE INTERCONNECTEDNESS OF THE BODY, MIND, AND SPIRIT, FOCUSING ON TREATING THE WHOLE PERSON RATHER THAN JUST THE SYMPTOMS.

4. **RECIPE**: A SET OF INSTRUCTIONS ON HOW TO PREPARE A PARTICULAR DISH OR CONCOCTION USING SPECIFIC INGREDIENTS AND TECHNIQUES.

5. **MEDICINAL PROPERTIES**: THE BENEFICIAL QUALITIES AND EFFECTS OF A SUBSTANCE, OFTEN RELATED TO HEALTH AND HEALING.

6. **PLANT MATERIAL**: THE RAW PARTS OF A PLANT USED FOR MEDICINAL PURPOSES, SUCH AS LEAVES, FLOWERS, STEMS, ROOTS, OR BARK.

7. **ALCOHOL**: A TYPE OF ORGANIC COMPOUND COMMONLY USED AS A SOLVENT FOR HERBAL TINCTURES, HELPING TO EXTRACT AND PRESERVE THE PLANT'S ACTIVE COMPOUNDS.

8. **EXTRACTION**: THE PROCESS OF DRAWING OUT OR SEPARATING THE ACTIVE COMPOUNDS OF A PLANT MATERIAL USING A SOLVENT, RESULTING IN A CONCENTRATED FORM.

9. **INFUSION**: A METHOD OF EXTRACTING THE MEDICINAL PROPERTIES OF PLANTS BY STEEPING THEM IN HOT WATER, OIL, OR ALCOHOL.

10. **DECOCTION**: A PROCESS OF EXTRACTING THE MEDICINAL PROPERTIES OF PLANTS BY BOILING THEM IN WATER OR OTHER SOLVENTS.

11. **DOSAGE**: THE SPECIFIC AMOUNT OF A HERBAL TINCTURE OR REMEDY RECOMMENDED FOR USE, OFTEN BASED ON FACTORS LIKE AGE, WEIGHT, AND SEVERITY OF THE AILMENT.

12. **INFUSED OIL**: A HERBAL PREPARATION WHERE PLANT MATERIAL IS STEEPED IN A CARRIER OIL (SUCH AS OLIVE OIL) FOR AN EXTENDED PERIOD, RESULTING IN AN OIL INFUSED WITH THE PLANT'S PROPERTIES.

13. **MACERATION**: THE PROCESS OF SOAKING HERBAL MATERIAL IN A LIQUID, OFTEN ALCOHOL OR OIL, TO EXTRACT ITS MEDICINAL QUALITIES.

14. **CARRIER**: A SUBSTANCE USED TO DILUTE A HERBAL TINCTURE OR REMEDY, ALLOWING FOR EASE OF APPLICATION OR CONSUMPTION.

15. **ALLEVIATE**: TO REDUCE OR RELIEVE THE SYMPTOMS OR SEVERITY OF AN AILMENT OR CONDITION.

16. **IMMUNE SYSTEM**: THE BODY'S DEFENSE MECHANISM RESPONSIBLE FOR PROTECTING AGAINST INFECTIONS, DISEASES, AND FOREIGN SUBSTANCES.

17. **DIGESTIVE SYSTEM**: THE BODILY SYSTEM RESPONSIBLE FOR BREAKING DOWN FOOD AND ABSORBING NUTRIENTS, OFTEN AFFECTED BY VARIOUS AILMENTS AND DISORDERS.

18. **NERVOUS SYSTEM**: A COMPLEX NETWORK OF NERVES AND CELLS THAT TRANSMIT SIGNALS BETWEEN DIFFERENT PARTS OF THE BODY, RESPONSIBLE FOR CONTROLLING BODILY FUNCTIONS AND RESPONSES.

19. **ANTIOXIDANT**: A SUBSTANCE THAT HELPS PROTECT THE BODY'S CELLS FROM DAMAGE CAUSED BY FREE RADICALS, WHICH CAN CONTRIBUTE TO VARIOUS AILMENTS AND DISEASES.

20. **ANTI-INFLAMMATORY**: A PROPERTY OR SUBSTANCE THAT HELPS REDUCE INFLAMMATION IN THE BODY, OFTEN ASSOCIATED WITH PAIN RELIEF AND IMPROVED OVERALL HEALTH.

SOURCES

1. BOOKS:

- "MEDICAL HERBALISM: THE SCIENCE AND PRACTICE OF HERBAL MEDICINE" BY DAVID HOFFMANN

- "THE HERBAL MEDICINE-MAKER'S HANDBOOK: A HOME MANUAL" BY JAMES GREEN

- "THE MODERN HERBAL DISPENSATORY: A MEDICINE-MAKING GUIDE" BY THOMAS EASLEY AND STEVEN HORNE

- "ROSEMARY GLADSTAR'S MEDICINAL HERBS: A BEGINNER'S GUIDE" BY ROSEMARY GLADSTAR

- "THE COMPLETE MEDICINAL HERBAL: A PRACTICAL GUIDE TO THE HEALING PROPERTIES OF HERBS" BY PENELOPE ODY

WEBSITES

- AMERICAN HERBALISTS GUILD (AHG): WWW.AMERICANHERBALISTSGUILD.COM

- NATIONAL CENTER FOR COMPLEMENTARY AND INTEGRATIVE HEALTH (NCCIH): NCCIH.NIH.GOV/HEALTH/HERBSATAGLANCE.HTM

- HERBAL ACADEMY: THEHERBALACADEMY.COM

- HERB RESEARCH FOUNDATION: WWW.HERBS.ORG

SCIENTIFIC JOURNALS:

- "JOURNAL OF ETHNOPHARMACOLOGY"

- "JOURNAL OF HERBAL MEDICINE"

- "JOURNAL OF ETHNOBIOLOGY AND ETHNOMEDICINE"

- "PLANTA MEDICA"

- "PHYTOTHERAPY RESEARCH"

ONLINE DATABASES

- PUBMED (WWW.NCBI.NLM.NIH.GOV/PUBMED)

- SCIENCEDIRECT (WWW.SCIENCEDIRECT.COM)

- JSTOR (WWW.JSTOR.ORG)